# WHEN PARENTS SAY NO

## SAY NO

### RELIGIOUS AND CULTURAL INFLUENCES ON PEDIATRIC HEALTHCARE TREATMENT

# Books Published by the Honor Society of Nursing, Sigma Theta Tau International

*When Parents Say No: Religious and Cultural Influences on Pediatric Healthcare Treatment*, Linnard-Palmer, 2006.

*Healthy Places, Healthy People: A Handbook for Culturally Competent Community Nursing Practice*, Dreher, Shapiro, and Asselin, 2006.

*nurseAdvance Collection.* (Topic-specific collections of honor society-published journal articles.) Topics offered are: *Cultural Diversity in Nursing; Disaster, Trauma, and Emergency Nursing; Gerontological Nursing; Health Promotion in Nursing; Implementing Evidence-Based Nursing; Resources for Implementing Evidence-Based Nursing; Leadership and Mentoring in Nursing; Maternal Health Nursing; Oncology Nursing; Pediatric Nursing; Psychiatric-Mental Health Nursing; Public, Environmental, and Community Health Nursing;* and *Women's Health Nursing.* 2006.

*The HeART of Nursing: Expressions of Creative Art in Nursing*, Second Edition, Wendler, 2005.

*Reflecting on 30 Years of Nursing Leadership: 1975-2005*, Donley, 2005

*Technological Competency as Caring in Nursing*, Locsin, 2005.

*Making a Difference: Stories from the Point of Care, Volume 1*, Hudacek, 2005.

*A Daybook for Nurses: Making a Difference Each Day*, Hudacek, 2004.

*Making a Difference: Stories from the Point of Care, Volume 2*, Hudacek, 2004.

*Pivotal Moments in Nursing: Leaders Who Changed the Path of a Profession*, Houser and Player, 2004.

*Building and Managing a Career in Nursing: Strategies for Advancing Your Career*, Miller, 2003.

*Collaboration for the Promotion of Nursing*, Briggs, Merk, and Mitchell, 2003.

*Ordinary People, Extraordinary Lives: The Stories of Nurses*, Smeltzer and Vlasses, 2003.

*Stories of Family Caregiving: Reconsideration of Theory, Literature, and Life*, Poirier and Ayres, 2002.

*As We See Ourselves: Jewish Women in Nursing*, Benson, 2001.

*Cadet Nurse Stories: The Call for and Response of Women During World War II*, Perry and Robinson, 2001.

*Creating Responsive Solutions to Healthcare Change*, McCullough, 2001.

*Nurses' Moral Practice: Investing and Discounting Self*, Kelly, 2000.

*Nursing and Philanthropy: An Energizing Metaphor for the 21st Century*, McBride, 2000.

*Gerontological Nursing Issues for the 21st Century*, Gueldner and Poon, 1999.

*The Roy Adaptation Model-Based Research: 25 Years of Contributions to Nursing Science*, Boston Based Adaptation Research in Nursing Society, 1999.

*The Adventurous Years: Leaders in Action 1973-1999*, Henderson, 1998.

*Immigrant Women and Their Health: An Olive Paper*, Ibrahim Meleis, Lipson, Muecke and Smith, 1998.

*The Neuman Systems Model and Nursing Education: Teaching Strategies and Outcomes*, Lowry, 1998.

*The Image Editors: Mind, Spirit, and Voice*, Hamilton, 1997.

*The Language of Nursing Theory and Metatheory*, King and Fawcett, 1997.

*Virginia Avenel Henderson: Signature for Nursing*, Hermann, 1997.

For more information and to order these books from the Honor Society of Nursing, Sigma Theta Tau International, visit the society's Web site at www.nursingsociety.org/publications, or go to www.nursingknowledge.org/stti/books, the Web site of Nursing Knowledge International, the honor society's sales and distribution division. Or, call 1.888 NKI.4YOU (U.S. and Canada) or +1.317.634.8171 (Outside U.S. and Canada).

# WHEN PARENTS SAY NO

## RELIGIOUS and CULTURAL INFLUENCES on PEDIATRIC HEALTHCARE TREATMENT

BY

LUANNE LINNARD-PALMER, EdD, RN, CPON

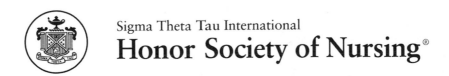

Sigma Theta Tau International
**Honor Society of Nursing**®

# SIGMA THETA TAU INTERNATIONAL

Editor-in-Chief: Jeff Burnham
Acquisitions Editor: Fay L. Bower, DNSc, RN, FAAN
Development Editor: Carla Hall
Proofreader: Jane Palmer

Cover Design by: Rebecca Harmon
Interior Design and Page Composition by: Rebecca Harmon

Printed in the United States of America
Printing and Binding by V.G. Reed & Sons

Sigma Theta Tau International
550 West North Street
Indianapolis, IN 46202

Visit our Web site at www.nursingknowledge.org/stti/books for more information on our books.

ISBN-10: 1-930538-30-8
ISBN-13: 978-1-930538-30-6

Library of Congress Cataloging-in-Publication Data

Linnard-Palmer, Luanne.
  When parents say no: religious and cultural influences on pediatric healthcare/ by Luanne Linnard-Palmer.
    p. ; cm.
  Includes bibliographical references and index.
  ISBN-13: 978-1-930538-30-6 (pbk.)
  ISBN-10: 1-930538-30-8 (pbk.)
  1. Children—Diseases—Treatment—Religious aspects—Handbooks, manuals, etc. 2. Children—Diseases—Treatment—Moral and ethical aspects—Handbooks, manuals, etc. 3. Pediatrics—Religious aspects—Handbooks, manuals, etc. I. Title.
  [DNLM: 1. Treatment Refusal. 2. Child Health Services. 3. Cultural Diversity. 4. Parental Consent. 5. Professional-Family Relations. 6. Religion and Medicine. W 85 L758r 2006]

RJ47.L56 2006
618.92—dc22

                                    2006016340
06  07  08  09  10  /  5  4  3  2  1

# DEDICATION

*This book is dedicated to my father, Howard W. Linnard.*

*A man of faith, truth, and courage.*

*I miss you every minute of every day.*

*Life is not the same without you.*

*Blessings to you in heaven.*

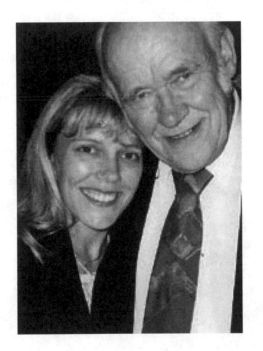

# Acknowledgements

Thank you, my precious family: **Logan,** you couldn't be more inquisitive, cuter, or understanding. **Christina,** your energy is inspiring and transformational—your little self melts my heart. **Evan,** you are so calm and supportive.

**Mom, Loren, Judith, Dean, Heather, Doug, Jessica,** and **Danielle:** Thank you for your faith in me.

**Susan Kools,** PhD, RN, professor of nursing: Without your support, gentle but powerful nudging, and belief in me, this book would not exist. Thank you for $2\frac{1}{2}$ motivational years during my postdoctorate studies at the University of California, San Francisco. I always loved coming to see you in your tranquil office. Your work ethic and professionalism inspired me.

Many thanks to **Dean Marty Nelson,** PhD, RN; **Dottie Needham,** PhD, APNP, RN, professor of nursing; and **Mary Ann Hauser,** MSN, RN, professor and director of undergraduate nursing at Dominican University of California, who gave me the time and encouragement to write.

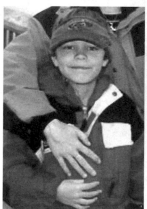
*Logan*

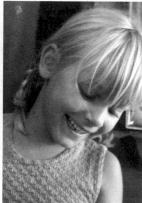
*Christina*

# About the Author

Luanne Linnard-Palmer has been a registered nurse for more than 21 years. She has worked extensively in adult and pediatric oncology. She is a tenured professor of nursing at Dominican University of California in San Rafael and works per diem as a pediatric clinical staff nurse at California Pacific Medical Center in San Francisco. Luanne was appointed chair of the Department of Nursing at Dominican in the fall of 2005. She received her BSN at Humboldt State University and her MSN and EdD at the University of San Francisco. Her postdoctoral studies were at the University of California, San Francisco under the direction of Susan Kools, PhD, RN.

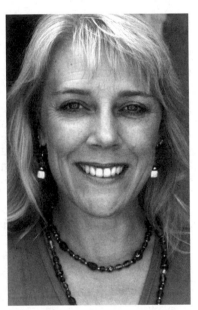

Luanne has two children, Logan and Christina, and has been married for 16 years. She plays the harp and thoroughly enjoys coming home from a stressful day of nursing, teaching, or administration to play classical and contemporary music, or play duets with her flautist brother, Loren Linnard. Luanne worships with her family at a small Episcopalian Church in San Rafael and is active on both the vestry and the Family Ministry Council. Raised a Methodist, she was influenced by her Christian Science mother and grandmother. Prayer, faith, and hope are important concepts in her daily life.

*The author, Luanne Linnard-Palmer*

# DISCLAIMER

The author's intention for this book is to accurately describe the perspectives and beliefs of various religious and cultural groups on medical care, as well as provide reports from lawyers, researchers, and academics—all without malice, judgment, or persecution. The information presented in this book came directly from current or past literature, media, Internet sources, or from direct quotes from personal communications received by the author. The perspectives shared by sources summarized for this book do not necessarily represent the views or religious beliefs of the author. The author did not intend to disclose personal perspectives on the critical topic of parental refusal or limitation of medical care for religious beliefs. Every attempt has been made to ensure the accuracy of the content of this book; however, any inaccurate reporting of religious beliefs, facts, quotes, or historical events is accidental and regrettable.

This book was not intended to pass judgment on the existence of divine, supernatural, or spiritual realms. The author, although a practicing Christian who includes prayer in her daily life, does not wish to pass judgment on religious decisions or beliefs of any kind. Rather, this book was written to give, as comprehensively as possible, a review of the phenomenon of treatment refusal. The intent behind this book is to offer guidance and a foundation for critical analysis for those involved in pediatric refusal situations.

# Table of Contents

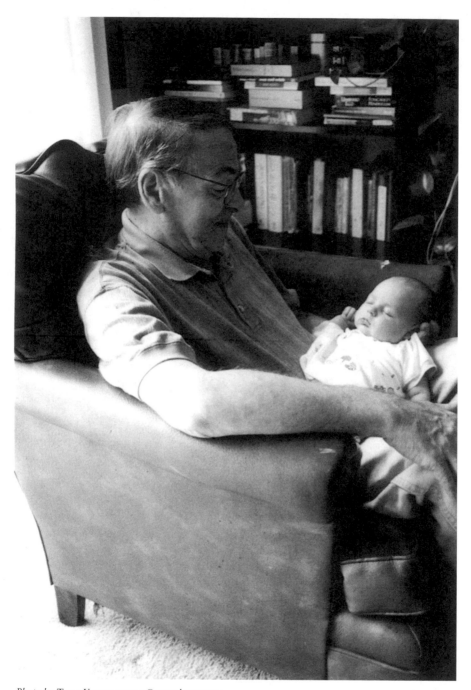

*Photo by Tracy Usman. usmans@tampabay.rr.com*

# FOREWORD
## by Lynn B. Clutter, MSN, RN, BC, CNS

Decisions about a child's healthcare treatment are often difficult when parents and professionals agree, but when they disagree, the conflict can present especially great challenges. Luanne Linnard-Palmer shares content about treatment refusal that is rarely discussed, but critically needed for healthcare providers in any setting that involves children.

Treatment refusal can bring ethical, moral, and spiritual dilemmas. Linnard-Palmer brings her talent for well-researched and thoughtful analysis to this book. She offers a meaningful exploration of complex and controversial situations. In clear and lucid descriptions, current findings are presented along with compelling case studies. Beyond that, state and national law content is interspersed while still maintaining a very readable style. *When Parents Say No* even includes an action plan, "Guidelines for Staff Facing Parental Refusal of Pediatric Treatment" (Appendix A).

Throughout my career and life, I have focused on *strengthening* the family, especially culturally and spiritually. I generally do not question parental authority. In writing this foreword, I want to avoid the erosion of any aspect of family strength. At the same time, I have to consider the mental, emotional, spiritual, and physical safety of children. What if a parent or healthcare professional makes a healthcare decision on behalf of a child that is, or could be, damaging? What happens when loving parents have deep-seated values and practices that clash with medical recommendations but are *not* dangerous to a child? Who and what should dictate care? When should the courts intervene? Linnard-Palmer directs our attention to these very situations to help us discover successful strategies of care.

Parents saying "no" to medical care is one of the most unsettling parts of decision-making in healthcare today. The choices can be extreme in any direction. State laws differ, and healthcare team approaches vary. This text gives examples of the "good, bad, and ugly" situations that may confront us.

With all our rhetoric for cultural sensitivity and comprehensive care, when it comes to working with parents who say "no," we have much to learn. This book presents examples that evoke emotion and question. Reading *When Parents Say No* caused me to contemplate my own core values about the issues presented. I hope that many will read its content and do the same. Indeed, many should. Working through ethical issues such as these can leave us with less emotion-based impulsivity in care and greater professional decision-making.

Answers are not spelled out, nor should they be. Solutions will be different in each case and in each state jurisdiction. Perhaps what is of greatest value is the personal growth this book evokes within the reader. I hope that, like me, readers will put aside their own biases and prejudices to consider the unique beliefs and practices that influence families to make decisions that may clash with decisions we consider optimal. I hope that healthcare providers will embrace the child within the family and within the religious or cultural community to honor lifestyle practices the family has chosen, but say "no" when the life of a child is in danger.

*Lynn B. Clutter, a maternal-child nurse since 1979, describes herself as a "family nurse." She is the author of* "Spiritual Issues in Children's Health-Care Settings," *in J.A. Rollins, R. Bolig, & C.C. Mahan (Eds.),* Meeting Children's Psychosocial Needs Across the Health-Care Continuum, *Austin, TX: Pro-Ed, 2005. She is currently working on her doctorate and is a mentee in the Chiron Mentoring Program.*

# INTRODUCTION

As immigration rates continue to grow, urban populations explode, and as church membership continues to increase at high rates, pediatric healthcare team members will encounter a wide array of cultural and religious beliefs on a more frequent basis. Some of these situations will go smoothly and some will not. Medical treatment refusal cases have the potential to result in child deaths, making it imperative that every member of the pediatric healthcare team be knowledgeable about how to react to treatment refusals and how to work with the family and clergy to create an environment for optimal outcomes.

Nurses, physicians, and related pediatric healthcare professionals are in a unique position to offer support to families who are experiencing the critical dilemma of wanting prayer in lieu of medical care, or wishing to limit medical care based on cultural or religious doctrine. Although the healthcare professionals involved may not agree with the application of parental cultural or religious beliefs on children's medical decision-making, and may proceed with securing state guardianship and mandated treatment, families deserve respect and a voice. They deserve the opportunity to explain their beliefs and preferences, alone or in the presence of their clergy or elder, when time is not dictated by the critical status of the child's condition.  They also deserve the opportunity to apply religious or cultural practices when safe and appropriate in the healthcare setting. Pediatric healthcare professionals can minimize the stress, fear, anxiety, and possible anger of family members by demonstrating an understanding of diverse beliefs and allowing time, whenever safe and possible, for each family member to disclose his or her concerns, belief systems and cultural practices.

Members of healthcare professions who encounter families of diverse cultural and religious backgrounds must be knowledgeable about legal and ethical principles, as well as the basic foundations of various religious doctrines. Healthcare professionals can be better prepared to participate in treatment decisions if they are well-versed in a variety of literature (and how to retrieve the literature) and are aware of the many viable perspectives on treatment refusal.

This book provides the historical background, legal implications and ethical concerns when families either limit or refuse traditional Western medical care based on their religious or cultural beliefs. Findings from recent ethnographic research are shared to provide examples of current refusal scenarios and to demonstrate the impact of the scenarios on all those involved. Numerous references, Web sites and current literature are offered to disclose the impact of this highly charged dilemma as well as examples of actual refusal situations. Practice guidelines are offered for the administration of safe interdisciplinary care during refusal situations.

*There are many reasons and influences that surround parental refusal of medical care for children, but religious and cultural beliefs are among the most profoundly influential.*

1

# OVERVIEW

Pediatric healthcare professionals administer care to children suffering from injuries, diseases, and disorders. When a parent refuses recommended treatment or sets treatment or diagnostic exam limitations, the situation can become strained and problematic. Few healthcare professionals know exactly what to do in such situations. The well-being of the child—even the survival of the child—is the ultimate concern of both parents and healthcare providers. Yet, who has the right to say what should and should not be done?

In many countries, there is great cultural value placed on the autonomy of parents' decisions for their children. These decisions include education, discipline, socialization, safety, and recreation. When it comes to medical decisions, it is generally understood that parents will supply competent healthcare.

Religion, beliefs, and spirituality are all important aspects of the lives of most Americans. According to the Gallup Poll (2006), 56% of the respondents indicated religion is very important to their lives; an additional 28% reported religion to be fairly important. Forty-four percent of the respondents described themselves as "born-again" or evangelical Christian; 62% reported that religion can answer all or most of today's problems. Seventy-three percent of American respondents reported they were convinced that God exists.

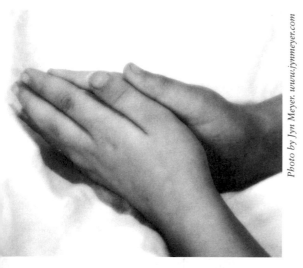

*Photo by Jyn Meyer, www.jynmeyer.com*

According to Clutter (2005), most people believe life has a spiritual aspect and God does indeed exist. The influence of these beliefs on family functioning is important to keep in mind as healthcare is delivered. As parents and children experience illness, trauma, disease, separation, and changes in life, professionals should keep in mind how important those beliefs may be (Clutter). When parents are faced with treatment decisions, including consenting for diagnostics and care, healthcare professionals should be ready to assess the family's religious beliefs and spiritual background and use this information to help all members of the family reach mutually acceptable and safe patient outcomes.

*According to Clutter (2005), most people believe life has a spiritual aspect and God does indeed exist.*

There are many reasons and influences that surround parental refusal of medical care for children, but religious and cultural beliefs are among the most profoundly influential. The focus of this book is on the various religious doctrines and cultural beliefs that influence parents' views and opinions on the application of traditional healthcare and on the corresponding legal, moral, and ethical processes that are initiated by pediatric parental refusal of vital treatments.

Most pediatric healthcare professionals report having encountered at least one refusal situation. Many indicate these ethical dilemmas leave a lasting mark on their memory and sometimes their career. Occasionally, the refusal scenarios go smoothly; other times, even with a multidisciplinary approach, the refusal scenario is highly charged and is perceived by those involved as a battle. After the last-ditch effort to incorporate a family's belief system into a Western model of traditional care, the healthcare team may determine that initiating legal proceedings is necessary to provide treatment. Sometimes parents lose guardianship of a child to the state for the time required to administer the mandated treatments. When this happens, the "battle" can become complex and volatile. However, court-mandated treatment is avoided whenever possible to keep relations smooth and the family on board for subsequent healthcare treatment.

Most pediatric healthcare professionals acknowledge they are ill-prepared to negotiate with families during treatment-refusal scenarios. Most of us, in fact, have minimal knowledge about the legal ramifications of such situations and also lack knowledge about religious doctrines and cultural beliefs that are important to many families.

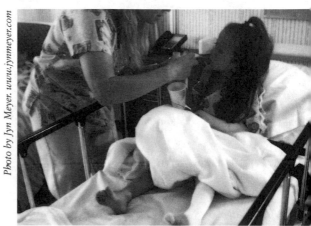

Photo by Jyn Meyer. www.jynmeyer.com

Pediatric healthcare professionals need access to resource materials to learn how to navigate through treatment-refusal scenarios. Knowing the legal influences, professional roles and responsibilities, and healthcare implications of religious beliefs and corresponding cultures is crucial. This book was written to provide members of pediatric healthcare teams—including those providing critical care, working in outpatient and home-care settings, and providing palliative and nontraditional or integral care—with a resource that can help them understand the complexity, diversity, and profound impact of pediatric treatment refusal.

Although a variety of professional experiences with pediatric treatment refusal have affected my career, the single episode that inspired my quest to learn about religious and cultural influences in parental treatment refusal involved an acutely ill boy suffering from profound anemia whose parents—both devout Jehovah's Witnesses—refused blood transfusion treatment for him. Their gravest concern was for the well being of his sould, particularly after the courts intervened and he was given the life-saving transfusion.

It is important not to belittle the impact of pediatric treatment refusal for all those involved. It is most distressing for the family if treatment wishes are not honored. It is also very difficult for the healthcare professionals involved to invest time-consuming and often morally distressing energy toward negotiations that frequently result in continued refusals. Most people want to avoid battles or disagreements over treatment decisions. This is not easy and often unavoidable, but negotiations for treatment, no matter how difficult, must be attempted. The goal is always the well-being of the child.

*The goal is always the well-being of the child, no matter what the process is to reach that goal.*

## DATA COLLECTION

This book is the result of a research study. Six broad questions guided the literature investigation, the in-depth interviews, and the ethnographic research studies that led to this book. These questions are listed below to clarify how the phenomenon of pediatric treatment refusal was first studied.

1) What are the historical events that have taken place over the last 100 years that have moved the perspective of a child from being "property without rights" of parents to having individual rights that supersede the constitutional rights of parents?

2) How have laws developed that provide healthcare professionals with the opportunity to seek and secure legally mandated temporary guardianship to administer lifesaving medical treatment or treatments to alleviate human suffering against the religious or cultural doctrines of families?

3) What ethical principles are at stake surrounding mandated treatment with or without the loss of guardianship? What are the ethical principles surrounding parents' authority to make decisions for their children?

4) What are the known examples of religious and cultural beliefs whose doctrines influence consideration of alternatives to, limitations, or refusal of basic Western healthcare and treatment modalities? What are exemplary illustrations of situations of refusal for each?

5) How does the situation of refusal and subsequent mandated treatment affect the child, family, and community of healthcare professionals? Is moral distress a frequently encountered outcome or a rare endpoint of extreme cases?

6) Which religious groups have doctrines or belief systems that influence healthcare treatment decisions? Where are they located? How influential are they, and what exactly do they propose? Which cultural groups have norms that influence parental healthcare decisions, and what are their beliefs?

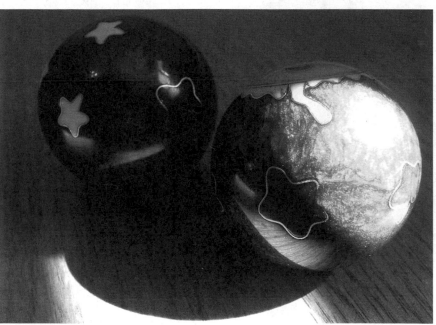

*Photo by Mark Iafrate. www.markiafrate.com*

The emphasis of the book is on the eminent need for healthcare professionals to acknowledge the presence of these groups in our current society and plan for interacting with group members to negotiate the best possible care for children. The number of religious groups and cultural groups that prefer prayer or cultural behaviors over Western medical care is unknown, but reports of the phenomenon are growing in the United States (Bromley & Melton, 2002). The intent of this book is to address a wide variety of religious and cultural groups without comparing their religious or spiritual frameworks, as each is separate and unique. All of the frameworks shared in this book are presented as accurately as possible using a variety of sources.

The value of love and concern for children is not in question throughout this book; rather the book is written to explain the phenomena of parents' refusal or limitation of treatment for their own children. Because it is often through love that parents apply religious or cultural beliefs, the family's concern for or commitment to the child is not in question. The concern is the outcome of the applications of these deeply held beliefs on the ultimate well-being of the child and his or her health state.

> *It is often through love that parents apply religious or cultural beliefs.*

# CASE EXAMPLES OF REFUSAL SCENARIOS

To understand the magnitude and impact of medical treatment limitation or refusal, it is important to first understand the situations that bring children to the healthcare arena. The following 11 cases provide brief examples of medical treatment refusal scenarios. The first six are from the author's clinical experiences, ethnographic investigations, or interviews; the last five are from recent media or Internet sources. The selected examples are stories or narrations shared by others through individual eyes and perceptions. Without a doubt, the following examples present a variety of perceptions depending on personal views, beliefs, life experiences, and memories of those involved.

## CASE ONE

An experienced registered nurse (RN) who specialized in pediatric hematology and oncology care arrived at work one Saturday morning in October at a large urban pediatric hospital to find an unusually large number of physicians, interns, residents, nurses, and family members standing in the hallway near the nurse's station. She received report and learned that a 4-year-old boy with sickle cell anemia, who was very ill, would be her patient that day. His blood work revealed severe anemia (a hemoglobin of 4.9 gm/dL), and he required an emergency blood transfusion. The parents refused the transfusion therapy, as they were devout Jehovah's Witnesses (JW). The pediatrician in charge of the child's care raised his voice slightly and informed the family and clergy present that there was no more time to negotiate alternatives, as the child was tachycardic and listless and

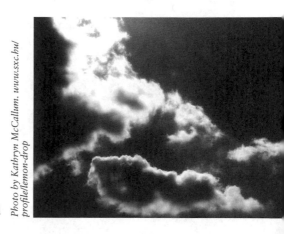

Photo by Kathryn McCallum. www.sxc.hu/ profilelemon-drop

could experience serious consequences from delayed therapy. The pediatrician then initiated phone calls to the hospital social services department, to hospital administrators, and to the county court representatives. He was able to secure temporary legal guardianship for mandated treatment for the time period required to administer the lifesaving blood transfusion therapy.

*The parents refused the transfusion therapy as they were devout Jehovah's Witnesses (JW).*

The parents were distraught but cooperated with the procedures. As the morning unfolded, the family shared with the nurse their beliefs about the possible consequences of the blood transfusion on the child's soul, his future relationship with God, and his chances of arriving safely in heaven (L. Linnard-Palmer, personal communication, October 15, 2004).

## CASE TWO

A 9-year-old girl was brought to a large urban pediatric hospital via helicopter after a neighbor notified county authorities of her medical condition. This young girl had stepped on a nail while visiting a national park with her family and had not been immunized for tetanus. She subsequently developed severe osteomyelitis from the puncture site in her foot up to her hip, with severe swelling, redness, pain, and loss of function. When the neighbor of the family noticed the condition of the child, she was being administered prayer within the home from faithful Christian Science practitioners. The child's medical condition warranted 6 weeks of intensive antibiotic therapy during her hospitalization. Unable to obtain the parents' written consent, the court agreed to grant temporary legal guardianship for the time period needed to treat the infection via a peripherally inserted central venous catheter. The family was present at the bedside and provided loving support to the child during her hospitalization (anonymous, personal communication, November 2003).

> *The court agreed to grant temporary legal guardianship for the time period needed to treat the infection*

## CASE THREE

A 14-year-old Islamic Muslim girl was recovering from a first-degree burn on her elbow from hot cooking oil that was spilled. The child had extensive surgical reconstruction, and her arm was slowing healing with a skin graft placed over the surgical site. While her extended family was visiting her at the bedside in a large Midwestern pediatric burn center, the medical team conducted bedside morning rounds to assess the child and her burn site. During this assessment, the family overheard the surgeon say that the pigskin graft was adhering well and leading to successful lower-tissue repair. Family members became very distraught that they had not been advised of the use of pigskin tissue. They demanded that the graft be removed. After failed negotiation attempts via family discussions about possible outcomes, the child was sent back to surgery, where the graft was removed. Afterward, the child experienced almost complete loss of function of her arm. Nevertheless, the family was appeased and satisfied that their spiritual and cultural requirements were upheld (anonymous, personal communication, October 2003).

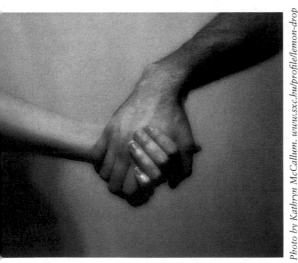

Photo by Kathryn McCallum. www.sxc.hu/profile/lemon-drop

## CASE FOUR

A teenage patient of an outpatient oncology unit had just been diagnosed with a rapid-growing lymphoma on her neck. The distraught family requested 3 to 5 days of comprehensive prayer with fellow parishioners of a large urban Christian church prior to what would possibly be an extensive stay in an inpatient pediatric oncology unit for high-dose induction chemotherapy. The oncologists tried to explain to the family that delaying the start of chemotherapy was risky because of the exponential growth measured on the young girl's tumor. Upon hearing that the oncologists wanted her to go directly to the hospital for treatment to be initiated that evening, the family took the child and left the clinic. The oncologist, fearful the family might not return or might choose to delay the onset of treatment by

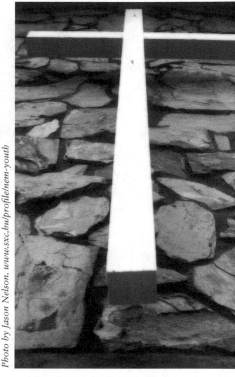

*Photo by Jason Nelson. www.sxc.hu/profile/nem-youth*

days, repeatedly telephoned the family to return. After hearing the telephone messages that legal guardianship for mandated treatment might be sought to ensure adequate treatment with a known probability of response, the family admitted the child for treatment the next day (pediatric oncology charge nurse, San Francisco clinic, personal communication, September 2003).

## CASE FIVE

A 10-year-old boy and his mother came to a busy emergency room (ER) of a large urban hospital. The child had had a moist, productive cough and a fever for more than 2 weeks. During medical history questioning, the mother reported the child had been successfully treated for a brain tumor at the age of 2. The ER personnel discovered the boy had a remarkably high serum white blood count (>300,000), which was a preliminary indicator of childhood leukemia. The mother became very distraught and explained to the ER staff that the child had suffered a great deal through chemotherapy and surgeries for the treatment of his brain tumor as a toddler. She said she could not bear to see him go through that again. If this was a true diagnosis, she announced to

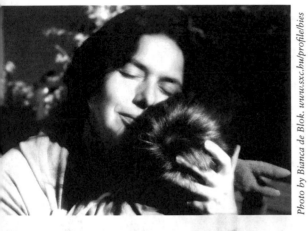

the ER staff, she would go down to rural Mexico, where her extended family was, and seek the assistance of a *curandero*. After being left alone behind a curtained-off ER bed while the staff contemplated what steps to take next, the mother and child left the ER against medical advice (AMA) and went home. After several unsuccessful attempts to contact the family at home, staff members were very concerned and subsequently notified social services, the hospital administrator, the hospital lawyer, and the county child protective services agency. Two days later, the social worker accompanied a law enforcement agent to the family's home and brought the child to the hospital for treatment. A court order for mandated treatment was required to ensure the child was treated for a diagnosis of leukemia. The mother was very upset. She stayed at the bedside at all times and documented every action of every staff member, stating she was going to sue. Although most difficult to deal with, the mother was allowed, and even encouraged, to stay, as she never physically obstructed the nurses, nor did she become belligerent again. The child responded to the cancer treatment and was released weeks later into his mother's care (anonymous, personal communication, October 2003).

## CASE SIX

A 2-year-old toddler was being treated for a new diagnosis of type 1 diabetes mellitus. The parents, faithful Muslims, requested the child receive only insulin that was human, not pork- or beef-based. The child experienced complications during his initial hospitalization and required intravenous therapy for dehydration and ketoacidosis. The heparin used for flushing his line was a low-dose anticoagulant used to keep the intravenous tubing patent and open. Unfortunately,

*The parents, faithful Muslims, requested the child receive only insulin that was human, not pork- or beef-based.*

the heparin was beef-based. Family members were very disappointed with the medical, nursing, and pharmacy teams, as they were not notified of the option of non-animal-based pharmaceutical products beyond the human insulin. The family was very vocal about its dismay and subsequently sought and received treatment at another hospital via a different pediatric internal medical team (ethnographic interview participant, personal communication, January 2001).

## CASE SEVEN

The Body, also known as The Body of Christ, is a small fundamentalist, Christian-faith group located in Attleboro, MA. The group consists of extended families living together in a communal lifestyle. They split from a larger Bible-study group in the late 1970s. Their faith-healing doctrine rejects traditional medical care, even disallowing the use of eyeglasses. Two infants were reported to have died within the closed community, both of whom were secretly buried in a state park in Maine. The cause of death for the two infants has not been disclosed in the media (New England Institute of Religious Research, n.d.).

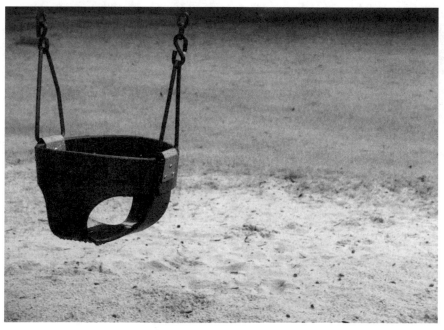

Photo by Kathryn McCallum, www.sxc.hu/profile/lemon-drop

## CASE EIGHT

In Florida, within a small evangelical Christian group, two children died between 1996 and 1998 as a direct result of the denial of traditional medical care. A 3-month-old choked to death because the family did not call for medical assistance (the parents were acquitted), and a 2-year-old died after being stung by 432 yellow jackets. The parents of the 2-year-old allegedly waited for 7 hours before calling the paramedics. When the paramedics arrived, the child had no pulse and was not breathing. The healthcare professionals involved in the child's resuscitation efforts determined the child had experienced great suffering. The parents were eventually charged with aggravated child abuse (Ontario Consultants on Religious Tolerance, n.d.).

*In Florida, within a small evangelical Christian group, two children died between 1996 and 1998 as a direct result of the denial of traditional medical care.*

## CASE NINE

Members of the End Time Ministries have been reported to have lost several church members in several states as a result of their exclusive belief in faith

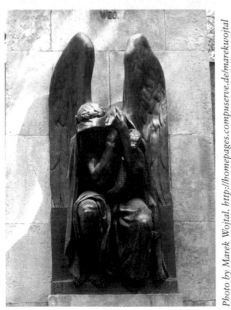

*Photo by Marek Wojtal. http://homepages.compuserve.de/marekwojtal*

healing. Five newborns died during home births (unattended by licensed practitioners), and two women died in 1990. The parents of a boy with a heart tumor were charged with child abuse when they refused an operation. The boy had lost approximately 30% of his weight, had kidney and liver failure, and suffered the consequences of long-term malnutrition. The same family lost a newborn child from massive hemorrhaging after the parents did not seek medical treatment (Ontario Consultants on Religious Tolerance, n.d.).

## CASE 10

Members of the Faith Assembly Church denied medical treatment for a 4-year-old with an eye tumor the size of the child's head. When law enforcement personnel assessed the situation, they found blood trails streaming along the walls of the home. These trails of blood were just the height of the young girl's head. Police discovered that the girl, who was nearly blind, used the wall to support her head and tumor as she walked room to room, leaving a streak of blood as she navigated between rooms. A neighbor reported the situation to the appropriate authorities, who then sought treatment interventions. Legal outcome of the situation was not disclosed in the report (Rick A. Ross Institute of New Jersey, n.d.).

## CASE 11

Parents of a comatose 10-year-old girl refused traditional rehabilitative treatment for their child, who had suffered irreversible brain damage following prolonged seizures after a near-drowning accident. The family, after many discussions through family conferences, was told further treatments would be required if any improvements of her condition were to be attained. The family adamantly expressed a desire to administer Chinese herbs and concentrated teas via her nasogastric tube. On several occasions, the nursing staff found the father administering solutions via the tube. After continuing investigations and negotiations, the medical team supported the parents' desires to co-treat the child with traditional Chinese medicine. The parents consented to further diagnostics and interventions once they felt their concerns were heard and respected and their cultural practices were accepted as a valuable source of healing for their child (anonymous, personal communication, October 2003).

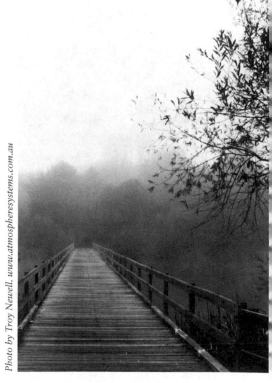

Photo by Troy Newell. www.atmospheresystems.com.au

## CASE 12

A 6-year-old boy in Bloomington, Indiana, died 3 months after child protection workers removed him from the care of his mother, an Indiana University professor who was born in China, and placed him with a foster family. The child had developmental problems and a variety of serious disorders, including a kidney condition that required the mother to catheterize him when he had trouble urinating. The pain of the procedure provoked the boy to bite and hit himself and others. Struggling to raise her son alone, the mother sought help from a social worker. During one visit, the mother mentioned that she had tied her son's hands with a terry cloth belt to keep him from hitting himself. The next day, police officers came to her home to pick up the boy, and he was placed with foster parents. While in state care, the boy's condition deteriorated, and he was hospitalized several times. He died April 1, 2004, one day after officials told the mother that her son would soon be returned to her (Evans & Trotter, 2006).

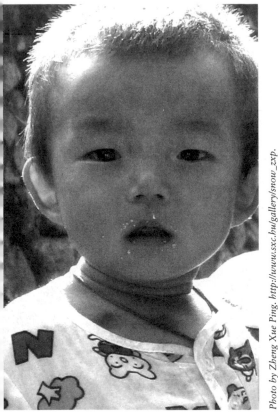

*Photo by Zheng Xue Ping. http://www.sxc.hu/gallery/snow_zxp.*

In 2002, the family traveled to Beijing, China, where doctors diagnosed the boy with renal tubular acidosis, a disorder that causes growth and developmental delays and painful urination problems (Murray, 2004). The Monroe County coroner, however, could not determine a cause of death, despite extensive toxicology tests and other examinations.

The child's parents filed a wrongful death suit against the state of Indiana and in July 2006, received a pretrial settlement of $350,000. The parents contended that the boy was wrongly removed from his mother's care because social workers did not understand her Chinese cultural heritage. Caseworkers did not understand Chinese mother-and-child bonding, the mother said (Evans

& Trotter, 2006). The boy was forced to eat American foods. When he was hospitalized, the mother was allowed to visit him with supervision but was forbidden from speaking to him in Chinese, the only language the boy knew (Trotter, 2004).

## CASE 13

I moonlighted recently at California Pacific Medical Center in San Francisco as a pediatric staff nurse. My patient-care assignment included a beautiful Russian Orthodox family whose 11-year-old son was recently diagnosed with acute lymphocytic leukemia, and he was receiving high doses of methotrexate chemotherapy. In addition, he was on high dose steroids with a side effect of severe weight gain, high blood sugars, and severe emotional mood swings. His mother, her husband, and the child's uncle held a prayer session at his bed after he had a long crying session about the despair he was feeling in losing his hair, gaining weight, and being separated from his beloved siblings and friends. I did not take part in the prayer session but gave them the time they needed to hold such a long session. I delayed my treatments and interventions and lab values to give them quiet time alone to pray. The child took part in the prayers and responded beautifully. He was quiet, serene, content, and felt loved afterwards. The event did delay my care but was well worth the response. He was emotionally stable after the session. (Linnard-Palmer, 2006)

# CASE REMARKS

These are but a few of the hundreds of cases taken from in-depth interviews and current literature. Not all of the above cases can be substantiated or confirmed, as not all Web-based sites can be deemed accurate in reporting a case. Some of the cases discovered in investigating sources for this book will never be brought to the public's eye, as they are resolved quietly between the family and healthcare team or between the primary physician and law enforcement, or they are not discovered by media reporters. There is no national registry or reporting mandate for these cases. The cases may or may not be reported as child abuse, and the parents may or may not be indicted for child abuse or neglect. The process of discovery and the follow-through, as well as the subsequent final outcome of these cases, can be quite varied.

*The cases may or may not be reported as child abuse, and the parents may or may not be indicted for child abuse or neglect.*

# PEDIATRIC HEALTHCARE, CHILD RIGHTS, AND ETHICS

## PEDIATRIC HEALTHCARE

Pediatric healthcare can be divided into five distinct areas:

1) Well-child care and health promotion education for normal growth and development.

2) Ongoing early disease and illness detection during routine screenings (vision, hearing, scoliosis, pediculosis, dental hygiene, child abuse and neglect, failure to thrive, and emotional distress).

3) Acute care of sudden illness needs, with interventions such as surgical procedures or antibiotic treatment.

4) Chronic care, in which a child is supported throughout childhood and adolescence during exacerbations of chronic conditions (cystic fibrosis, cancer, or diabetes).

5) Palliative, hospice, or comfort care when aggressive treatments are no longer indicated, and the focus is on symptom management and support for end-of-life care.

Each of these care areas can be influenced by parents' perspectives, beliefs, and cultural norms. Each experience is unique for every family, and each family has unique needs.

Pediatric healthcare is complex in that a child may be seen by more than one traditional pediatrician and by specialty pediatricians. The child also may encounter advanced practice nurses—such as clinical nurse specialists, nurse practitioners, community health or public health nurses, and school nurses—all of whom deliver care in diverse settings. A child might be followed by a social service specialist, a developmental specialist, an academic support person, or some other specialty-care group that provides family support and resources. All of these disciplines may find their services are influenced by the family's religious beliefs or cultural norms. It is imperative that these groups be aware of how belief systems can be an influence on all areas of family functioning and a child's life.

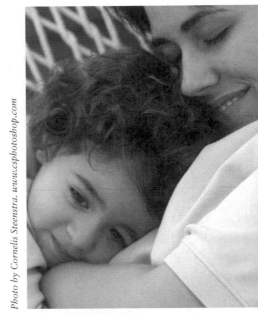

*Photo by Cornelis Steenstra. www.csphotoshop.com*

## HISTORY OF CHILD RIGHTS IN THE UNITED STATES

The concept of child rights is relatively new in American history. In the United States, animals were legally protected from cruelty before children received those rights. It was not until the early 1900s that children were legally protected against work injuries and laws were established that limited the hours and conditions of children's labor. According to a health science professor at Dominican University of California (personal communication, 1996), a New York lawyer was the first American to pursue legislation for child rights. The story goes that in 1905, the lawyer came upon a child chained to a fence while both parents were at work. From the parents' perspective, chaining the socially isolated child to the fence was the only way to keep him "safe" (never mind the exposure to the elements and acts of human cruelty). Greatly moved by this case, the lawyer immediately went to work to secure children's legal rights to protection from harm.

*Parents have the right to consent to care for their dependent children; they do not have a co-equal right to refuse care for their dependent children.*

Parents have the right to autonomously raise their children. The United States Constitution specifies that parents have the right to raise their children in relation to discipline and education. The Constitution does not, however, endow parents with the right to withhold essential medical interventions or screenings on the grounds of religious or cultural beliefs. Thus, the dichotomy between healthcare professionals and parents with distinct and influential beliefs occurs because of the desire to provide care for children while respecting parental autonomy. The United Nations Committee on the Rights of the Child monitors states' compliance with international guidelines and laws passed by the United Nations. This work is overseen by the Office of the United Nations High Commissioner for Human Rights (see www.ohchr.org/english/bodies/crc/). These guidelines endow all children with reasonable and appropriate rights, including medical care; however, the UN database of articles does not specifically address medical treatment refusal by parents.

Flannery (1995) describes how several U.S. Supreme Court decisions have supported what is considered a constitutional right to "bring up children," yet another Supreme Court decision held that parents have a constitutional right to make medical decisions for their children "absent of finding of abuse or neglect" (p. 9).

In 1944, the U.S. Supreme Court ruled "the right to practice religion freely does not include liberty to expose … a child … to ill health or death. Parents may be free to become martyrs themselves, but it does not follow that they are free … to make martyrs of their children before the children reach the age of full and legal discretion when they can make that choice for themselves" (Prince v. Massachusetts, 1944).

Adults have the right to refuse medical treatments because they have been granted self-determination. Children, however, are not considered autonomous and can neither give informed consent nor refuse treatment. Courts will at times override parents' decisions to refuse treatment based on the state child abuse or neglect law (Fox, 1990).

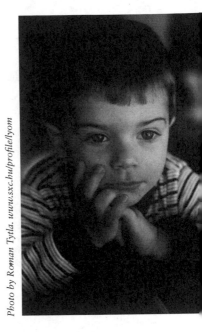

Historically, parents' rights over their children's lives were considered absolute. Now, in relation to withholding necessary medical treatment, parents have limits. According to Fox (1990), "A county court in New York ruled that when parents' religious beliefs interfere with a child's right to live, the child's right is paramount, and the religious doctrine must give way" (p. 136). The right to refuse medical treatment for children is obviously a very complex phenomenon that has evolved throughout history.

There are three legal bases for the right of an adult to refuse treatment:

1) the right to freedom from nonconsensual invasion of bodily integrity, embodied in the informed consent doctrine and the law of battery;

2) the constitutional right of privacy; and

3) the constitutional right to freedom of religion (Rhodes & Miller, 1984).

These are widely accepted legal perspectives used when the person of concern is an adult. When the person of concern is a child, these laws do not apply. Under certain situations, when competent adults have made healthcare decisions for minors that deviate from expected medical treatment application, courts have found it necessary to view the state's interest as outweighing that of the treatment decision-maker and have ordered treatment to take place. This seems to be in direct conflict with the three legal bases for refusal as described above. Yet, when the minor is in a life-threatening situation, the courts have overridden the decision-making rights of the parent or guardian. "Because decision-makers have an obligation to act in the best interests of the minor or incompetent adult, they must provide necessary (medical) treatment" (Rhodes & Miller, 1984, p. 216). Discretion to decline treatment is limited to situations where the treatment is elective or not likely to be beneficial. The duty to provide necessary treatment to minors is reinforced in all states by legislation concerning abused or neglected minors. This duty facilitates state intervention to provide needed assistance.

*Yet, when the minor is in a life-threatening situation, the courts have overridden the decision-making rights of the parent or guardian.*

The state's authority to act as guardian for children who are unable to make healthcare decisions is deeply entrenched in the history of 20th-century laws. Via physician requests, state authorities may seek to protect a child by moving the child from his or her present custodian to another and intervene on the minor's behalf to ensure the necessary medical treatments are given. This is the case when the custodian, a parent or legal guardian, has been deemed unreasonable in his or her refusal to supply medical treatment based on religious or other grounds (Humber & Almedar, 1998).

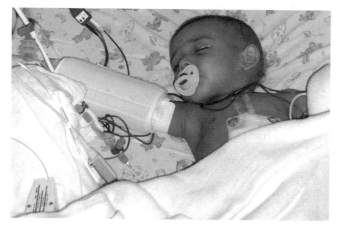

*Photo by Farrukh Usman.*

According to the Committee on Bioethics of the American Academy of Pediatrics (1988):

> The boundary between parental freedom in child rearing and the interest or even basic rights of the child is unclear. The limits to parental decision-making for children are uncertain, but it is widely accepted that parents generally will make decisions that do not directly threaten the welfare of their children. Tradition, social forces, and the belief systems shape the limits of acceptable nurturance or parental imperatives and privileges, and even of physical force used in the discipline of children. These, of course, change with time. However, the constitutional guarantees of freedom of religion do not sanction harming another person in the practice of one's religion, and they do not allow religion to be a legal defense when one harms another. (p. 169)

## ETHICS

The application of ethical principles must be considered when discussing parental treatment decisions leading to either the refusal or limitation of children's basic healthcare needs. Fox (1990) identified four main ethical principles at stake when withholding or limiting medical treatment for children. These principles include:

1) **Autonomy:** The insistence that all people have intrinsic worth and therefore self-determination, including both the right to decide medical treatment and religious freedoms.

2) **Beneficence:** Basic healthcare assumptions that include promoting welfare as well as "acts of mercy and kindness."

3) **Non-maleficence:** Considered a greater obligation than beneficence, referring to not inflicting evil or harm.

4) **Justice:** The concern of fairness or impartiality.

Long-standing ethical doctrines pertaining to parental rights in the care of their children include parental autonomy, parens patriae, best interest, and substituted judgment (Cushing, 1982). Each of these important doctrines has an influence on treatment limitation or refusal.

**Parental autonomy** is a protected right or personal liberty offered within the United States. Pediatric healthcare professionals, in general, respect parental autonomy. Parents usually are the experts with their children. They are usually the ones with the greatest love and attention toward their children. Healthcare professionals honor the strength of this relationship and include parents whenever possible in a child's care. Professionals will not interfere as long as abuse, neglect, or suffering are not present.

It is within the scope of practice for pediatric healthcare professionals to offer parenting guidelines and support so that a family is cohesive and well-adjusted to the social circumstances and culture in which that family lives. It is, nevertheless, an important professional duty to assess for effective parenting skills and identify early family crises or situations where a child might be placed at risk. It then becomes the legal duty of a pediatric healthcare professional to intervene and possibly report the consequences of the risk (such as abuse or neglect) to the appropriate authorities.

**Parens patriae, Latin for "parent of the country,"** is a state's right and duty to protect children and to act as the decision maker when needed. This right means healthcare providers are required to report all cases of child abuse or neglect. Once reported to state authorities, decisions are in the hands of those authorities (i.e., child protective agencies).

**Best interest doctrine** is a requirement of a court to consider subjective and objective evidence when evaluating what is best for a minor's welfare. Several data sources can be used, including neighbors, church members, school officials, and so on.

**Substituted judgment** is a court's determination, on behalf of an incompetent individual, of what choice the individual would make if the individual were competent. This is considered more subjective than the best interest doctrine.

*Pope John Paul II reportedly described forcing someone to violate his or her conscience as the most painful blow inflicted on human dignity. He believes it may even be worse than killing.*

The application of these ethical principles and doctrines might be needed when parents refuse medical treatment. One concern is the interference of the courts to become a decision-making body, thereby leaving a family, specifically the parents, without the power to decide what is right for their child. This leaves the parent unable to direct the child's life, including applying cultural norms and practices or religious doctrines or beliefs. The second concern when applying ethical principles and doctrines encompasses determination of what is truly best for the child, which could mean taking away the right of the parents to adhere to their religious doctrines. This conflict is seen in the writing of Fox (1990): "The result of the violation of a deeply held, long-standing religious conviction can be devastating. Pope John Paul II reportedly described forcing someone to violate his or her conscience as the most painful blow inflicted on human dignity. He believes it may even be worse than killing" (p. 138).

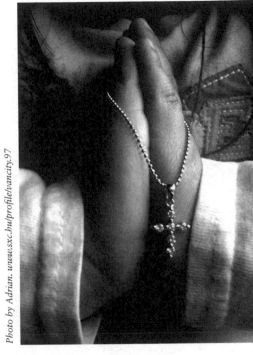

*Photo by Adrian. www.sxc.hu/profile/vancity.97*

There can be no doubt how powerful this ethical dilemma is, both for family members, who want to adhere to their religious faith or cultural norms, and members of the healthcare team, who must live with the consequences of their actions—not just specifically their consciences, but also the consequences on the child and family. Both legal and ethical doctrines shed light on these dilemmas and allow all people involved to begin to understand what the dilemma encompasses and how to move toward an ethical conclusion or an ethical answer.

According to Catlin (1997), the phenomenon of treatment refusal or limitation of treatment in the pediatric population places members of the healthcare team in a "classical ethical dilemma" (p. 289). Two competing harms have been described by Catlin as: (1) the articulated harm of a child in a critical condition that may be worsened by withholding medical treatment; and (2) the more explicated harm that takes place when a parent's decision-making is overruled or legally contravened. Healthcare team members, including nurses, have been taught to respect personal differences. Diverse

*Participation in an ethical dilemma between divergent frameworks in healthcare situations can lead to personal distress for the nurse.*

races, cultures, ethnicities, and religious frameworks are aspects of client care that nurses consider. Participation in an ethical dilemma between divergent frameworks in healthcare situations can lead to personal distress for the nurse. Nurses, for instance, have been encouraged to advocate for patients and families, yet the petition for legally mandated temporary guardianship to enforce medical treatments may be perceived as in direct conflict with the notion of parent and family advocacy.

Much has been written about the advocacy role inherent in the practice of nursing. Yet, some of the most crucial advocacy situations carry a risk factor, particularly in relation to the care of children. Can one be a professional advocate when the basic support for religious preferences and application is prohibited? Many questions remain unanswered, and neither the medical nor the nursing science literature demonstrates much inquiry into this debate. According to Catlin (1997):

> Nurses recognize that one of the greatest joys that exist in parenting is sharing with one's children the values of family traditions and culture. Christians baptize their children, Jews circumcise their males, Muslims fast at Ramadan, and Hindus have ceremonies of anointing with oils and spices, and rarely do nurses interfere with closely held, faith-based customs. (p. 289)

Being a child advocate for activities and practices that cause no harm or human suffering is easy. Being a child advocate when a parent's application of religious or cultural practices leads to withholding essential healthcare is difficult or may be contrary to safe practice. Glover and Rushton (1995) succinctly describe this difficult ethical debate.

> We may claim certainty about medical facts, or about what our faith traditions require as a way of avoiding difficult discussions and decisions. If we resort to unilateral decision-making by professionals or parents, we risk cutting moral

> dialogue short and seriously misconstruing our shared obligations to our children. (p. 5)

Because philosophical analysis rather than empirical inquiry has guided much of the current activity in bioethics, research in clinical practice is greatly needed. The methods of ethnographic research support the inquiry of the impact of treatment refusal on the parent, child, family, clergy, and healthcare professional's experiences. Much of this book is dedicated to the presentation of ethnographic research methods that were used to explore the impact of parental medical-treatment refusal, with or without loss of guardianship, on the experiences of all involved.

# LEGAL IMPLICATIONS

## COLLABORATING WITH CHILDREN ON TREATMENT DECISIONS

A question contemplated by members of pediatric health science disciplines is whether or not children have the capacity to participate in collaborative decision-making concerning health-care and treatment decisions. Research has shown that when children's developmental stage, not solely their chronological age, is considered, their input can be a sincere influence on treatment decisions. This is a critical thought when parents are refusing medical treatment or wishing to limit medical treatment based on their own religious beliefs, which may or may not be shared by the child. Pediatricians and pediatric nurses should assess the child's ability to give input and value his or her verbalized wishes as a component of the treatment trajectory.

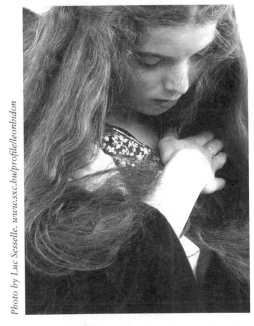

Photo by Luc Sesselle. www.sxc.hu/profile/leonbidon

## INFORMED CONSENT

To illustrate a child's ability to give input into treatment decisions, note the following example. A nine-year-old boy—nearing his 10th birthday—named Tommy refused treatment for a recurring brain tumor. Tommy had been diagnosed with a rapid-growing supratentorial brain tumor at the age of seven. At that time, the family had requested treatment be delayed in order to have a team of church members assemble to pray for their son's healing. Reluctant to support this delay, the pediatrician and pediatric neurosurgeon had been able to convince both parents to consent to treatment and had persuaded the influential grandparents to offer their support during the initial treatments. At the time of the recurrence near Tommy's 10th birthday, the parents willingly consented to further treatment. Tommy, however, vehemently refused to undergo surgery and chemotherapy again. The child's quality of life was affected by his initial treatments three years prior. Tommy articulately expressed his desire not to experience chemotherapy and surgical interventions again. Ultimately, he did receive treatments for this second episode of tumor re-growth, but the discerning medical team gave Tommy time to express his fears, concerns, and wishes. As it turned out, his concerns were not associated with the actual treatments but were focused on whether or not he would receive adequate symptom management and relief from nausea, pain, and sleep disturbances leading to chronic fatigue.

*Patients have the right to know all options for treatments, all available diagnostic options, and the risks and benefits associated with each.*

The American Academy of Pediatrics (AAP) published an initial policy statement in 1976 that articulated the legal concept of "informed consent" in pediatric medical practice. Historically, the authority to make medical decisions lay solely in the hands of physicians. Now, in response to continuing complex social changes, physicians must ask permission and consent from their patients, as the patients have the right to decide. Patients have the right to know all options for treatments, all available diagnostic options, and the risks and benefits associated with each. Parents also have a right to this knowledge when children require medical treatment, but they do not have the right to withhold life-sustaining or lifesaving treatments based on their cultural or religious beliefs nor do they have the right to cause harm.

## ASSENT

The concept of assent has been formalized. The AAP Committee on Bioethics states that children should participate in decision-making *commensurate with their development,* providing assent to care whenever reasonable. The term "assent" refers to a child's formal statements of contribution during decision making. The age of assent has been estimated as being about 12 (Foreman, 1999), although various institutions may have varying policies on the minimal age, including having children as young as seven participate in family conferences or treatment decision-making.

According to the AAP Committee on Bioethics (1995), physicians should seek parental permission in most situations. They must focus on the goal of providing appropriate care and be prepared to seek legal intervention when parental refusal places the patient at clear and substantial risk. When parents refuse "appropriate care," pediatricians should seek consultative assistance and use judicial determinations only in rare or unusual circumstances. Because only patients who have appropriate decisional capacity and legal empowerment can give their informed consent, assent of an underage child should be sought whenever appropriate and considered during treatment decisions.

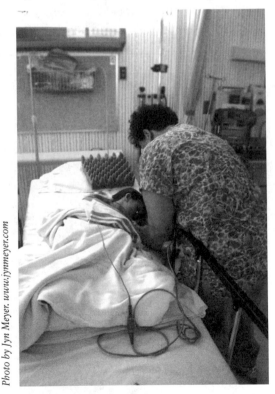

Photo by Jyn Meyer. www.jynmeyer.com

## PARENTAL PERMISSION

In order for physicians to perform diagnostics, interventions, and medical services for a child, they must legally acquire parental permission. Permission is sought in two ways: the verbal agreement dictating permission from the parent after a discussion on the processes, risks, and benefits, as well as the alternatives available; and by a witnessed signature of the parent or legal guardian. There are times during administration of emergency care that verbal permission is sought and a signature is acquired later, but this is not ideal. It is imperative, when both parties are able, to secure verbal permission and a signature on a consent form, to avoid the potential of litigation or confusion about the necessary medical interventions. Diagnostic evaluation, blood product transfusion, and minor or major procedures require parental (or legal guardian) permission by way of informed consent.

If parents are not willing to sign a consent form because of religious or cultural beliefs, state courts in this country have historically been willing to hold that religious convictions and beliefs, in and of themselves, are not a true defense to criminal liability for those families whose religious practices exclude medical care (Monopoli, 1991). In these cases, the physician may need to seek court interventions in the way of temporary guardianship to provide needed diagnostics and interventions. Full parental permission, support, and consent are ideal and smooth the process of providing healthcare to children.

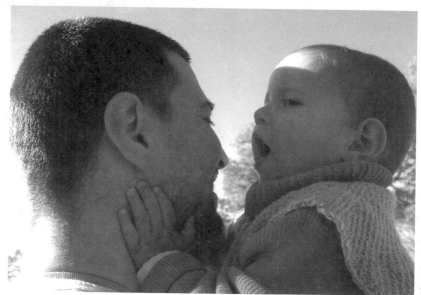

*Photo by Vedrana Bosnjak. www.artmobil.hr*

# LEGAL PERSPECTIVES OF TREATMENT REFUSAL

*Governing bodies such as individual state legislatures create laws that protect the well-being of children. These protective laws are under the umbrella of child abuse and neglect laws and are created to prevent human suffering, harm, and death due to parental acts of omission and commission.*

Refusal has been defined by Appelbaum and Roth (1983) as the "overt rejection by the patient, or his/her representative, of medication, surgery, investigative procedures, or other components of hospital care recommended or ordered by the patient's physician" (p. 1296). Refusal of medically needed healthcare is no longer deemed an obscure phenomenon, but rather has recently become the focus of literary attention.

When a parent refuses basic medical treatment deemed to be lifesaving, the healthcare team members may need to contact social workers, hospital officials, and possibly child-protective agency representatives to petition juvenile or family court systems to obtain legally mandated temporary guardianship (Anderson, 1983). Time should not be spent during the critical period of treatment decision-making attempting to change parental refusal for consent to treatment by asking the parents to give up their beliefs (Quintero, 1993).

According to Swan (1997), U.S. parents do not have a First Amendment right to abuse or neglect children. There is always the possibility of criminal liability when parents refuse medical treatment for their child based on religious or cultural beliefs. Swan states that only a minor fraction of cases of children dying because of treatment refusal based on religious doctrine have resulted in actual prosecution.

As discussed earlier, the three American Constitutional bases for the right to refuse treatment for competent adults—freedom from nonconsensual invasion, right of privacy, and the constitutional right to freedom of religion—do not apply to children who are of nonconsenting age or who are unemancipated minors. Governing bodies such as individual state legislatures create laws that protect the well-being of children. These protective laws are under the umbrella of child abuse and neglect laws and are created to prevent human suffering, harm, and death due to parental acts of omission and commission.

According to research conducted by Seth and Swan (1998): "When faith healing is used to the exclusion of medical treatment, the number of preventable child fatalities and the associated suffering are substantial and warrant public concern. Existing laws may be inadequate to protect children from this form of medical neglect" (pp. 625-629). Child fatalities in faith-healing sects were reviewed by Seth and Swan, and the probability of survival for each case was estimated based on survival rates expected of children who receive medical care for similar disorders. Their findings indicate that withholding medical care and exclusively using prayer leads to poorer health outcomes. Seth and Swan highly support laws that ensure safe, adequate, and thorough medical care for all children.

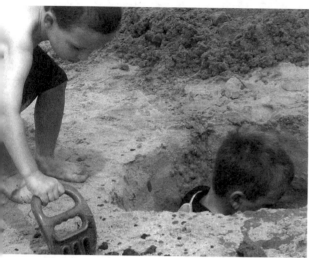

*Photo by Fay Bower.*

Legal actions come in several forms. Courts, for instance, will generally allow parents to refuse extraordinary care when the minor is in a coma or considered terminally ill. In one such case, the Supreme Judicial Court of Massachusetts allowed a "no code" status to be put in place for a child younger than one who was considered terminal. Another case involved a New Jersey father who was allowed by that state's Supreme Court to extubate his irreversibly comatose daughter (Rhodes & Miller, 1984). Courts do not intervene in situations where the families are offered unorthodox treatments or when the benefits do not clearly outweigh the risks. For example, in the case of an 11-year-old with a severely deformed arm, the Washington Supreme Court refused to authorize amputation of the child's arm. The parents had refused the surgery, but the physicians felt amputation was medically warranted.

Five reasons for courts to override a patient's right to refuse medical treatment have been noted within several U.S. laws:

1) preservation of life when the patient's condition is curable;

2) protection of the patient's dependents, especially minor children;

3) prevention of irrational self-destruction;

4) preservation of ethical integrity of healthcare providers; and

5) protection of the public health and other interests.

In relation to minors, state laws generally focus on protecting the minor's welfare (Rhodes & Miller, 1984). In relation to children making consensual decisions about their healthcare, the United Kingdom's Children's Act of 1989 considers 16-year-olds to be capable of making their own treatment decisions (Purssell, 1995). There have been instances when U.S. physicians in pediatric oncology practice have granted autonomous treatment decisions to minors who were 17 years old, regardless of parental refusal or support for the child's cancer treatments. At 17 years of age, minors can become legally responsible for their healthcare treatment decisions by seeking (and receiving) legal emancipation.

*At 17 years of age, minors can become legally responsible for their healthcare treatment decisions by seeking (and receiving) legal emancipation.*

The patient under the age of 18 presents an increasing dilemma for U.S. healthcare professionals. Considered legally incompetent, by definition, adolescents "are legally unable to give informed consent for treatments or to unilaterally refuse medically indicated treatments" (Lantos & Miles, 1989, p. 461). Two distinctly different situations can occur in the care of adolescents. They may align their religious or cultural beliefs with the parents and request withholding or limiting certain medical treatments, or they may request to be treated against the parents' belief systems. Four principles have been described by Lantos and Miles (1989) concerning these types of situations:

1) The physician's ethical obligation to act in a beneficent manner justifies emergency treatment.

2) The right to privacy when considering sexual or reproductive health leads to dilemmas in including parental input.

3) The concept of a mature minor allows the healthcare team to sidestep the legal presumption of incompetence and permit treatment decision-making.

4) The right to exercise religious freedom in decisions to refuse treatment is sometimes considered.

All four of these guiding principles can leave medical professionals in a quandary. Emergency treatments, although logical and lifesaving, may indeed be acts against the belief systems of the family. If adolescents seek information or treatments for sexual or reproductive health issues while requesting privacy, and parents have made their cultural or religious beliefs clear to the care providers, conflicts may arise. If parents are vocal about their wish for medical treatment for a mature minor, yet the minor does not want to be treated, healthcare providers find themselves in a conflict of interest between parties. The right to refuse treatment based on religious freedom may create a conflict for the healthcare provider when the adolescent may not fully comprehend the health risks. Solutions come from careful consideration of the wishes of all parties while applying the law.

Legal doctrine pertaining to adolescents refusing medical treatment continues to be unclear and may rest with the perceptions of the physician. The court may look to the physician for guidance when endorsing treatment refusal. The two questions judges tend to ask physicians are:

1) Is there a medical need?

2) Is there a medically feasible response?

If both questions are answered affirmatively, judges may then provide the legal means to administer treatments. Quality of life is not considered for such decisions; rather, if a lifesaving treatment is available, it must be undertaken (Paris, 1982).

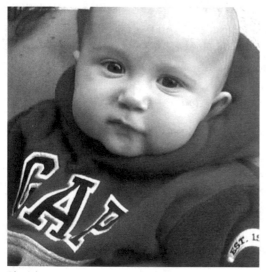

From personal observations and conclusions drawn from interviews, it is apparent the physician and all members of the healthcare team should include school-age children and adolescents in treatment decision-making whenever possible.

*Photo by Fay Bower.*

*Children in this country are still being martyred on the altar of their parents' religious beliefs. Parents cloaking themselves in the First Amendment and its free exercise clause are denying their children medical treatment and those children are dying.*

2

# FACTORS THAT INFLUENCE PARENTAL REFUSAL

## HISTORICAL INFLUENCES OF TREATMENT REFUSAL

History provides a context for viewing the development of health sciences and how the field became what it is now. Considering the first medical record was not developed until 1920, it is clear how far medicine and related fields have developed in a relatively short time. Now, the medical record is one of the most important tools for communication between professionals, for tracking patient progress, as a source for research, and for prevention of litigation. Where were we before that time?

Treatment refusal within pediatric practice is not readily traceable. Information became available after the first medical records were created and subsequently during the securing of child rights. No absolute way has been found to trace the accurate history of healthcare refusal scenarios or to document the historical development of influential church doctrines. Nevertheless, influential court decisions around parental refusal or limitation of medical care over time were found in the literature from varied sources. These court decisions are summarized in the following chronological list:

| 1878 | Courts limit the right to certain religious practices when those practices impinged on the rights of others. |
|------|---|
| 1903 | The First Amendment to the Constitution for religious freedom does not give the right to withhold medical care from a child (People v. New York, Peirson, 1903) |
| 1944 | "The right to practice religion freely does not include the liberty to expose ... a child ... to ill health or death" (Prince v. Massachusetts, 1944). |
| 1951 | In all cases documented to date, courts have ordered that children receive transfusions when medically indicated, even if their parents refuse. Courts may grant mandatory treatment orders over the phone within 15 minutes of a petition, as most hospitals have 24-hour legal consultation available (Fox, 1990). |
| 1962 | U.S. courts upheld an adult patient's right to refuse blood on the grounds of protection of individual choice (even to the point of loss of human life). |
| 1975 | The U.S. Department of Health, Education, and Welfare set forth regulations to implement the Child Abuse Protection and Treatment Act of 1974, giving definitions and a requirement that a state include a prayer-treatment option. |
| 1982 | Baby Doe Case, with issues centered on the withholding of duodenal atresia surgery from a Down syndrome baby and court-ordered surgery. |
| 1983 | The U.S. Department of Health and Human Services (formerly the Department of Health, Education, and Welfare) removed the prayer-treatment exemption and defined child neglect to include denial of medical treatment. This was accomplished by new regulations, which provide that nothing in the federal rule should be viewed as prohibiting or requiring a finding of child abuse or neglect when parents participate in their religious beliefs and withhold medical treatment. The regulation provides a proviso that |

supports the application of medical care in the face of neglect, regardless of the presence of an exemption, in that the exemption will not limit an agency or service from providing required medical care.

| | |
|---|---|
| 1984 | Amendment to the Child Abuse Prevention and Treatment Act included wording that all newborns must receive maximal life-prolonging treatment (Baby Doe regulation). Federal legislation was enacted to prevent neglect of handicapped infants. |

| | |
|---|---|
| 1988 | Neonatologists expressed concern to the U.S. Supreme Court over Baby Doe regulation. The question of whether or not each case should go to court for review received intense scrutiny. |

*The right to practice religion freely does not include liberty to expose the community or the child to communicable disease or the latter to ill health or death.*

Where are we now? The most recent position of the American Academy of Pediatrics (AAP) is that exemptions should continue to be re-evaluated and revoked as needed to ensure safe measure for ill children. Although the AAP's major concern is treating the child, the academy's position includes demonstrating sensitivity to and allowing all voices to be heard.

According to Monopoli (1991):

> The right to practice religion freely does not include liberty to expose the community or the child to communicable disease or the latter to ill health or death. ... Parents may be free to become martyrs themselves. But it does not follow they are free, in identical circumstances, to make martyrs of their children before they have reached the age of full legal discretion when they can make that choice for themselves. It has been almost 50 years since the Unites States Supreme Court wrote these presumably unambiguous words in Prince v. Massachusetts. Yet children in this country are still being

martyred on the altar of their parents' religious beliefs. Parents cloaking themselves in the First Amendment and its free exercise clause are denying their children medical treatment and those children are dying. (pp. 320-321)

# IN THE NAME OF RELIGION: HISTORICAL INFLUENCES TO LEGAL EXEMPTIONS

Religious exemptions from child abuse laws were first passed in 1974 by all U.S. states as a reaction to a federal government mandate. U.S. federal authorities decided they would not allocate federal funds for any state for child protection programs unless religious exemptions were provided. Eleven states had exemptions in place by the end of 1974. Within 10 years, all 50 states had an exemption in place. Some states (Arizona, Washington, Illinois, and Connecticut) met these federal requirements by providing religious ex-

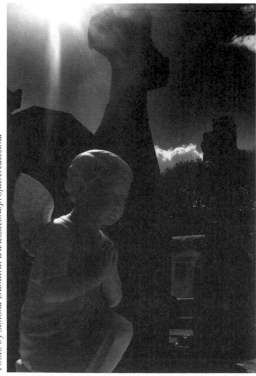

*Photo by Simona Dumitru. www.sxc.hu/profile/createsima*

emptions to Christian Scientists only. One by one, states have changed their exemptions over the years to allow a greater ability to prosecute for withholding medical care as a form of child abuse, even though earlier the federal government promoted exemptions. At the time of publication of this book, all U.S. states except Iowa and Ohio can prosecute for manslaughter when a child dies from parental treatment refusal based on religious doctrines (Children's Healthcare is a Legal Duty [CHILD], n.d.).

In 2000, Swan reported 41 U.S. states had religious exemptions from child neglect or child abuse charges, while 31 states allowed a religious defense from criminal charges. Two states, Ohio and Iowa, still have religious exemptions from prosecution for manslaughter, while Delaware and West Virginia continue to allow religious defenses for murder charges. Arkansas alone allows for religious defenses against capital murder.

> States with a religious defense to child endangerment, criminal abuse or neglect, and cruelty to children include Alabama, Colorado, Delaware, Georgia, Idaho, Indiana, Iowa, Kansas, Louisiana, Maine, Minnesota, Missouri, Nevada, New Hampshire, New Jersey, New York, Ohio, Oklahoma, South Carolina, Tennessee, Texas, Utah, Virginia, West Virginia, and Wisconsin. (Swan, 2000, p. 8)

The timeline goes as follows: Congress' 1974 directive required states receiving federal money for child abuse and prevention programs were to have exemptions for parents who substituted prayer or healing for medical care. This directive was rescinded in 1983, 9 years later, as most states had already enacted religious exemptions. "Then in 1996, Congress seemed to reverse itself in the Child Abuse Prevention and Treatment Act, saying there was no federal requirement that a child must be provided any medical service or treatment against the religious beliefs of the parent or legal guardian" (Janofsky, 2001, p. 1).

In 2001, Congress reauthorized the federal Child Abuse Prevention and Treatment Act (CAPTA), requiring states receiving federal money for programs against child abuse have laws that require parents to provide needed healthcare services. However, CAPTA allows "statutory exemptions" for parents with religious objections.

Clearly, the history around the U.S. government's commitment to protect children is confusing and may have been highly influenced by organized religions lobbying for protection against prosecution. Swan (2000) asks a succinct question:

> Why, in the 21st century, is this situation allowed to continue? It may be because the United States remains reluctant to fully acknowledge children as right-bearing persons. The public and its lawmakers aren't ready to give children a constitutional right to healthcare. While states do require par-

ents to provide their children with the necessities of life, they don't always require that children receive adequate health-care. And every state, at one time or another, has passed laws allowing parents to withhold, on religious grounds, some forms of medical treatment. Religious exemption laws create two classes of children. One is entitled to preventive, diagnostic and therapeutic healthcare because their parents have a legal duty to provide it. The other, those in faith-healing sects, have no right to immunizations, prophylactic eye drops, health screenings and, depending on the reach of the religious defense in the criminal code, no right to medical care for illnesses unless and until a state agency becomes aware of their needs and obtains care by court order. (p. 9)

*Children have rights too, and parents have certain rights which end when they intrude too far into a child's right to live.*

According to the CHILD Web site, www.childrenshealthcare.org, 48 states continue to have religious exemptions for immunizations and metabolic testing for newborns. Delaware, Illinois, Kansas, Maine, Massachusetts, New Jersey, and Rhode Island allow exemptions for testing for lead levels in a child's blood. California, Colorado, Massachusetts, Michigan, Minnesota, and Ohio have statutes that allow students with religious objections to be excused from studying about human diseases.

In 1988, the national office of the American Civil Liberties Union (ACLU) made a statement in regard to the presence of religious exemptions:

> Children have rights too, and parents have certain rights which end when they intrude too far into a child's right to live. ... The parent's right to bring up the child in the way the parent thinks best—an important right ... ends at the point in which the parents' actions endanger the lives of kids. ... There cannot be in our view a religious exemption no matter how sincere a parent's belief. (Massachusetts Citizens for Children, 1992)

In 1983, the U. S. Department of Health and Human Services (USDHHS) no longer mandated states include exemptions for religious doctrines that influence healthcare decisions for children. Rather, the USDHHS requires states to provide medical treatment in their definitions of child neglect (Swan, 1997). In fact, Congress added a statement to the Child Abuse Prevention and Treatment Act Amendments of 1996 that requires parents to provide needed medical services for a child, even against their religious or cultural beliefs, and imposed a moratorium on USDHHS requiring changes in revoking religious exemption laws (Swan).

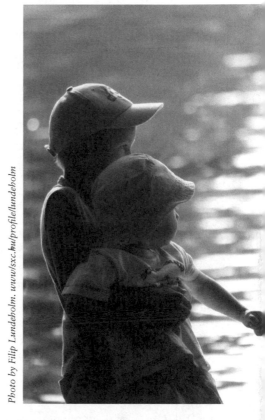

Photo by Filip Lundeholm. www/sxc.hu/profile/lundeholm

Many states have exemptions to their child abuse and neglect laws for spiritual treatment. These exemptions do not mean the courts will not intervene on behalf of the child, especially when the child is in a life-threatening situation. This troublesome conflict within the legal system continues to be addressed in the courts. The states' authority to act as guardian for those children who are unable to care for themselves continues to be deeply entrenched in the law (Neely, 1998).

At the time of publication of this book, Iowa has presented legislation to repeal the religious defense to felony child endangerment and manslaughter (CHILD, 2006).

States with religious defenses to severe crimes include:

1)  Iowa and Oho, with religious defenses to manslaughter

2)  Delaware and West Virginia, with religious defenses to murder of a child

3)  Arkansas, with religious defenses to capital murder

4)  Oregon, with religious defenses to homicide by abuse (CHILD, n.d.).

Organized religious groups can be quite influential regarding the writing and passing of state laws. Historically, U.S. courts have found it appropriate to order medical treatment over parents' objections when treatment is necessary to prevent the child from dying. Most courts have held that intervention is also appropriate when necessary to prevent "grievous harm" to a child (Dwyer, 1996).

# Clergy Responsibility and the Law

Most churches have a leadership group responsible for the oversight of the structure and function of the religious organization. In some religious organizations, clergy are responsible for finances and daily operations. In others, clergy are a separate constituent whose sole responsibility is to teach, model, and apply church doctrine, leaving the day-to-day responsibility of church function to a church governing body. Whatever the structure, clergy can be seen as highly influential to the church community in the application of religious doctrine. Most states see this position as one of power and influence and therefore may hold the clergy member responsible for the outcomes of religious-doctrine application. Parents, on the other hand, may deviate from their church's beliefs, doctrines, or teachings and proceed on their own faith path.

The legal responsibility of leaders of churches whose doctrines and teachings affect health-related decisions is an influencing factor in medical treatment refusal. Great legal commentary exists as to the level of legal responsibility the clergy should have when a child is harmed or dies from a delay or abstinence of traditional medical treatment based on religious doctrine. Discussions can be found in the literature concerning what is termed "clergy malpractice." According to Dodes (1987), a "typical clergy malpractice action alleges conduct such as improper pastoral counseling, intentional infliction of emotional distress, inadequate teaching or intentional interference with contractual relations, and the plaintiffs sue as representatives of the injured or deceased child" (p. 166). On the other hand, the First Amendment to the U.S. Constitution provides that "Congress shall make no law respecting an establishment of religion or prohibiting the free exercise thereof." The very presence of the First Amendment language demonstrates that there is no complete separation of church and state and gives rise to involvement of sorts (Dodes, 1987).

In actions alleging church negligence, the plaintiffs are often unable to proceed with their litigation because of the constitutionally protected nature of church conduct under U.S. federal and individual state constitutions. Although the controversy would be justifiable if the defendants were private individuals, churches have been absolved from civil litigation by virtue of the doctrine of separation of church and state. "Policy which supports the judicial rule of preventing adjudication of a negligence action against a religious organization should not serve to insulate faith healers from liability by preventing legal recourse to families of children being sacrificed in the name of religion" (Dodes, 1987, pp. 166-168). It is important to emphasize that many religious institutions and members believe in prayer for healing. The difference in the problematic groups is that they do not at the same time believe in receiving medical treatment.

The distinction between *belief* and *conduct* is interesting to note. Religious *belief* affecting children may qualify for First Amendment protection, whereas religious *conduct* may not. If a church is immune from civil liability, it may be because the medical treatment refusal for a child was considered to be *secular conduct*, which can be regulated by law, versus *secular beliefs*, which cannot (Dodes, 1987).

The following is an essay that was provided as a creative and thorough viewpoint from an experienced pastor on the ethical dilemmas that face those in a position of power over a congregation. The essay focuses on the polarity of viewpoint and behavior when one's main objective is to apply religious or cultural beliefs.

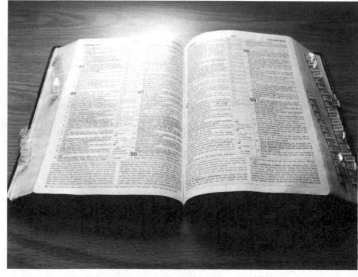

*Photo by Gerson Robles. www.sxc.hu/profile/gershom*

*Few of us would argue against prayer as an adjunct to other therapies.*

## ACTION AND BELIEF

To understand ethics within any society, the concepts of action and belief must first be discriminated, followed by their counterparts of faith and behavior. Our democracy bases its conception and perpetuation upon certain "inalienable rights," among which are life, liberty, and the pursuit of happiness (Declaration of Independence). Whatever we *believe* with regard to these rights, we must insist that all citizens act in such a way that these rights are not abridged for any.

Absolute individual freedom exists only in isolation—the vacuum where all human interaction has ceased to exist. But where we propose society, human concourse, and interaction, absolute individual freedom recedes from the world of action into the realm of thought. We are, and shall always be, free to *believe* whatever we wish, whatever our emotions or reason dictate; but we must *behave* in a manner that ensures as much freedom as possible for each member of that society.

For instance, we may *believe* in human sacrifice; we may not, however, act on that belief. If murder is permitted, society deviates and dissolves; both belief and action are abrogated.

The ethical axiom is: Freedom of belief (or thought) does not presuppose freedom of action. (Immanuel Kant: "I ought implies I can; but I can does not necessarily imply I ought.") Belief and actuality are not identical. For religious reasons, I may *believe* the world to be flat. That faith, however, does not alter the external reality of a round world, nor may I act on that faith. Again, I may wish to posit the absence of the effect of gravity on my body. Through my prayers and deep meditation, I *believe* that I can emancipate myself from all effects of gravity. However, if I step into empty space outside my 32nd-story hotel window, the actuality of gravity will destroy both my belief and my life. I was sincere in my faith; I was also sincerely wrong in my action.

Medical procedures that involve either the infusion or the extraction of blood (leeches, transfusions, even incisions) are understood by some religious groups as biblically forbidden. While we may argue the philosophical and theological accuracy of these sects' interpretations, we may not proscribe their beliefs. But we may enforce that any action on those beliefs, particularly toward those over whom religious practitioners hold actual or psychological authority, must be strictly regulated, particularly if it contravenes any adherent's physical or psychological health.

Society continually makes distinctions between belief and action within our legal system in many areas outside the field of medical practice and ethics. For example:

1) Advocates of nudist colonies may believe and preach the benefits, spiritually and physically, of worshiping the sun by living as much as possible without clothes. The law recognizes the right of nudists to believe such tenets. However, no nudist child is permitted to attend school in his or her "natural state" (without clothes); no nudist adult is permitted to walk the streets or work in their preferred "natural state."

2) Countless academics and nonacademics have believed in the beneficial use of psychohallucinogenic drugs (one needs only to mention Dr. Timothy Leary, the former Harvard University professor of psychology, who experimented on himself and his students, publicizing his advocacy for the possession and use of LSD). Consistently, our society via our legal system proscribes against the medicinal or recreational possession, sale, or ingestion of any psychedelic preparation. No matter how intensely a parent may believe in the salutary efficacy of mood-altering drugs, he or she may neither use these drugs nor allow them to be used by children.

3) Steroids may become the drug of choice for athletes who believe that their ingestion will enhance their competitive performances. Although athletes and coaches both believe in the benefits of steroidal therapy, their actions in using them are strictly forbidden.

4) Some religious communities believe that demon possession is the etiology of mental illness. Therapies to alleviate the possession often include purging, flagellations, burning (of suspected body parts, e.g., the genitalia in the case of sexual perversion), or the administration of other kinds of pain to draw out and frighten away the evil spirits. These beliefs and faiths are guaranteed by the U.S. Constitution and Bill of Rights; acting upon those beliefs, however, is not tolerated within our social structure.

5) Many individuals and groups within the conservative and fundamental Christian religious traditions believe prayer alone is capable of effecting physical and mental cures. These groups believe that pharmacological or surgical intervention disrupts the mind-body-spirit continuum. Some believe that prayer alone limits Divine Providence in its action within that cosmos it created. If we presume it logical to believe God speaks through prayer, is it not logical to assume some Deity's activity directs the minds of modern medical researchers as they discover newer and more effective means to recapture and ensure health? Are not prayer (God's gift) and medical research and discovery (also God's gift) to be seen as two sides of the same Divine coin?

Questions arise, particularly from medical practitioners, regarding the efficacy of prayer. Classical theologians (St. Augustine, Karl Bart, and others) agree with the following concerning prayer: Prayer surrounds situations and individuals with beneficial, soteriological (saving/wholeness-producing) atmosphere within which relaxation and healing may be promoted.

Such prayer depends upon the free will of that person who is the object of intercessory prayer. Human free will is never suspended by Deity simply because other people have decided to intercede (to interfere, in some interpretations) in another person's life. Only an individual's "openness" and willingness to receive make the beneficial aspects of prayer possible.

Few of us would argue against prayer as an adjunct to other therapies. We understand the psyche's ability to think through difficult situations and, through relaxation and meditation, stimulate the body's ability to "breathe through" intense pain. Natural childbirth presupposes just this ability.

When we work with the weakest and most vulnerable within our society (children, those who are emotionally and mentally limited, those with diagnosed psychiatric problems, and cognitively impaired elders), the conscientious intervention by healthcare professionals on their behalf is ethically demanded and morally mandated. For the preservation of mankind, the health and freedom of all who live within it, responsible *behavior*, regardless of *belief*, is required. That is the role of government and the legal system; it is also our moral obligation. We do not proscribe *belief*; we do, however, demand salutary *behavior*.

Dr. Dwight E. Conrad, OSL

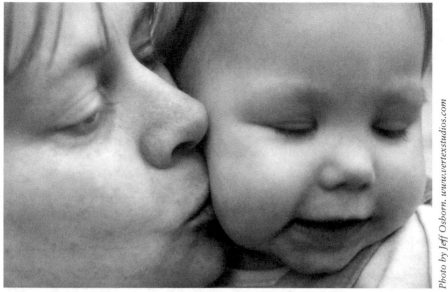

*Photo by Jeff Osborn. www.vertexstudios.com*

# LEGAL EXEMPTIONS TO SPECIFIC TYPES OF HEALTHCARE TREATMENTS

In the United States, some states have kept legislation in place to allow exemptions from routine health screening, immunizations, and other very specific, health-related childhood interventions. According to Dr. Rita Swan, founder and president of CHILD, state and federal legislatures have historically given parents "religious rights to endanger their children" (Swan, 2000.) She points out that exemptions from preventive and diagnostic measures continue to exist, even though these measures are widely known to prevent childhood diseases, injuries, and illnesses. She cites, for example, the statistic that 48 states continue to have religious exemptions from routine childhood immunizations. Mississippi and West Virginia are the two states that require all children to receive immunizations, with no consideration or exemption for religious doctrines or beliefs. Furthermore, the majority of states continue to have exemptions for newborn metabolic testing. These tests detect the presence of an actual or potential disease in the neonate for which there may be interventions to prevent illness, blindness, mental retardation, or even death (Swan, 2000).

A common prevention for severe disease, and sometime blindness, in newborns is the administration of antimicrobial eye drops or ointments in the

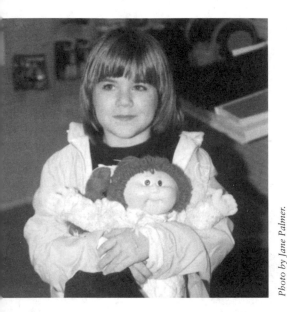

Photo by Jane Palmer.

eyes of all newborns. Chlamydia and gonorrhea are two of the microbial infections that can be easily prevented by the routine instillation of eye drops for all neonates. Iowa, Minnesota, Colorado, and Michigan all have religious exemptions for families, so they can refuse eye prophylaxsis for their neonates based on religious beliefs. According to Swan (2000), California, Colorado, Michigan, Minnesota, and Ohio statutes include religious exemptions for routine health screening offered as preventive healthcare in public schools. "California, Connecticut, New Jersey, and West Virginia have a religious exemption from hearing tests for newborns. California, Colorado, Massachusetts, Michigan, Minnesota, and Ohio have statutes excusing students with religious objections from even studying about disease in school, and California has a religious exemption from tuberculosis testing of public school teachers" (p. 7).

Delaware, Illinois, Kansas, Maine, Massachusetts, New Jersey, and Rhode Island have religious exemptions for the routine screening of children for lead poisoning (Swan, 2000). Lead poisoning is often a silent disorder where a child's blood levels of lead slowly rise without gross detectable signs. When the level reaches a certain point, many body systems can be affected and massive neurological damage, seizures, coma, and death can occur. Lead poisoning continues to be a plague. Many countries continue to have lead substances—gasoline, construction paint, ceramic paints, and industrial exposures—present in soil, food, and cookware. Children who are not screened but are at risk may suffer several disorders and symptoms including anemia, nausea, and failure to thrive.

According to the American Academy of Pediatrics:

> In the United States, the constitutional guarantee of protection of religious practice from intrusion by government has

been used by some religious groups to seek exemption from legislature or regulatory requirements regarding child abuse or neglect. Certain groups have succeeded in obtaining exemption from reporting or prosecution for child abuse and neglect including medical neglect, in more than three quarters of the states. There are now statutes in 44 states which contain a provision stating that a child is not to be deemed abused or neglected merely because he/she is receiving treatment by a spiritual means, through prayer, according to the tenets of a recognized religion. (International Cultic Studies Association, n.d., para. 5)

Educational exemptions also exist for children of religious parents who believe certain topics may be harmful or conflict with their beliefs. According to Dwyer (1996), most states exempt certain types of educational instruction received in nonreligious (public) schools. These topics include sex education and instruction in health and family life education.

California's Education Code provides a general exemption:

Whenever any part of the instruction in health, family life education, and sex education conflicts with the religious training and beliefs of the parent or guardian of any pupil, the pupil, on written request of the parent or guardian, shall be excused from the part of the training which conflicts with such religious training and beliefs. This provision includes personal moral convictions within the meaning of religious training and beliefs. (Dwyer, 1996, p. 1352)

Believing one is immune to prosecution for failure to provide medical treatment may be one of the most influential reasons parents choose to apply religious beliefs in lieu of medical care. They may believe no matter what happens, they have the legal right and state-sanctioned support to continue to withhold medical care since exemptions continue to be in place.

*Believing one is immune to prosecution for failure to provide medical treatment may be one of the most influential reasons that parents choose to apply religious beliefs in lieu of medical care.*

*When parents refuse to cooperate with the "standard"*
*expected of hospitalized patients and their families, for*
*whatever reason, healthcare team members can become*
*derailed and uncomfortable.*

3

# REASONS FOR TREATMENT REFUSAL

## OVERVIEW

Religious or cultural influences, although the basis of this book, represent just two of the many identified reasons why parents "say no" to traditional Western medical care. The frequency of treatment refusal for children in general is well-documented in the literature, media, and court proceedings. The exact frequency of the phenomenon of medical treatment refusal and subsequent loss of temporary guardianship of minors is unknown. Interviews with a number of nurses and physicians who have worked extensively in the field of pediatrics revealed there are many stories of treatment refusal based on religious frameworks, culture, and other reasons. Examples of loss of guardianship following treatment refusal are found less frequently, demonstrating that refusal situations are often handled without the need to obtain state court intervention. No current literature describes an accounting of treatment refusals, but as far back as 1983, Applebaum and Roth discussed how pediatric treatment refusals are well-documented, yet numbers are not accounted for.

Between 1975 and 1995, 172 children reportedly connected to 18 religious sects died because of parental objection or refusal of medical intervention (Swan, 1997). As cited by Seth and Swan (1998), of the 172 children identified by referral or record searches who died during that time, 140 fatalities were from conditions for which medical care could have provided a 90% survival rate; 18 likely would have had a survival rate in the area of 50%; and all but 3 of the rest would have likely had some clinical benefit as a result of the application of traditional medical care.

There are numerous powerful reasons behind parental decisions to refuse or limit medical treatment. The following list was condensed from health science and related literature of the past 21 years.

1) Religious frameworks concerning preference for prayer over traditional medical treatments or prior to any traditional medical care were found nationally and internationally.

2) Religious frameworks concerning limits on interventions such as various blood and blood product transfusion therapies, specialized diet therapies, or diagnostics have been found across America.

3) Ambiguous consenting procedures by healthcare professionals seeking parental approval and signature for medical treatments, diagnostics, or other procedures can lead to refusal to sign consent forms. Often, healthcare providers try to rush the process for obtaining consent for diagnostics, treatments, transfusions, or surgeries, leading parents to refuse or delay consent. This rush is often related to the hectic interdisciplinary schedule of pediatric hospital departments.

4) Conflicting or ambiguous sources of information regarding treatment decisions can occur. Because of the vast array of technology, it is not uncommon for parents to seek second or third opinions, which can then delay consent or treatments.

5) Influences on access to sophisticated medical technology can lead to fears, confusion, and delays in treatment consent.

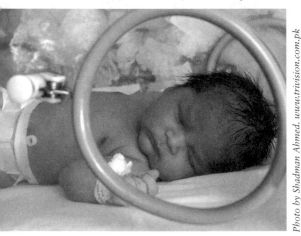

*Photo by Shadman Ahmed. www.trivision.com.pk*

6) Pressures during the treatment decision-making time frame can occur. Some religious or cultural practices warrant counsel; by church elders, high-level church representatives, or tribal leaders, which in turn causes treatment delays.

7) Conscientious objectors to medical care or treatment exist. Some people simply do not trust or wish to apply modern, standardized medical care. Many in this category are not affiliated with any particular cultural or religious group. Some may believe the procedures are overlapping, or repeated measures are just not warranted. Sometimes they are right and sometimes they are not. This mistrust may add to the confusion.

*Conscientious objectors to medical care or treatment exist. Some people simply do not trust or wish to apply modern, standardized medical care.*

8) Use of alternative medicine modalities rather than Western medical practices has become commonplace. With the rising number of Americans who use complementary, alternative, or integrative treatments, parental desires to apply various nontraditional healing methods are escalating.

9) Parental relationships with other siblings can become strained or compromised, and the sacrifice of family life (quality of life) during the demands of care for the child requiring treatment may be perceived to be too great. In other words, families may say "No" to a complex and expensive treatment for one child, so that the quality of life of the family as a whole is not changed or is minimally impacted.

10) Cost in dollars, loss of employment compensation, or inability to maintain employment during care for the ill child can cause parents to refuse treatment.

11) Mental capacity of parents during treatment decisions may influence consenting procedures or treatment decision-making. Illiteracy, lower educational levels, and poor comprehension abilities can influence whether or not a parent readily consents for medical treatments.

12) Pressures and emotional turmoil during treatment decisions may be too great.

13) Mental capabilities of children concerning treatment decisions may influence parents' treatment decisions.

14) Issues concerning best interest for the child may influence consenting procedures.

15) Concerns of quality of life for the child after complex medical treatments with few known positive outcomes may influence parental decisions.

(Information summarized from Overbay, 1996; Paris & Bell, 1993; Rhodes, 1999; Ruccione, Kramer, Moore, & Perin, 1991).

There are probably more reasons that can be identified, as family constellation, structure, educational level, function, and decision-making power differ for each unique family system. The current scientific literature clearly demonstrates how our nation's healthcare system is arranged for parents to bring in their ill child; consent to prescribed diagnostic exams, pharmaceuticals, treatments, and surgeries; and allow the healthcare system to make the treatment decisions. Healthcare providers have efficient routines on which they rely on a daily basis. Most do not want these routines disrupted. Western medical systems are fast-paced, with practitioners accustomed to cookie-cutter precision and too busy to be concerned with individual needs. When parents refuse to cooperate with the "standard" expected of hospitalized patients and their families, for whatever reason, healthcare team members can become derailed and uncomfortable. Pressure on the parents to cooperate can lead to future dissonance and departure.

*The emotional impact of having an ill child is monumental.*

The emotional impact of having an ill child is monumental. Parents are often not in the right state of mind or emotionally prepared to consent to imminent medical interventions for their child. There is no one solution for this situation, as early interventions for most childhood illnesses produce better outcomes. Yet, tragic consequences can occur when treatments are performed without full parental involvement and consent and interventions are carried out against the family's beliefs, convictions, or principles. Critical concern based on data for each situation is needed.

*Not all religions have had children become gravely ill or die due to prayer in lieu of medical care, nor do all church members follow the doctrines or teachings of particular religions that promote withholding medical care for their members.*

4

# OVERVIEW OF RELIGIOUS DOCTRINES

## INTRODUCTION

Several religious frameworks support refusal or limitation of medical care and treatments or prayer as the larger component of healing. In the data collected for this book, 31 separate churches that adhere to these limit or refusal frameworks were identified, covering an historical time frame of 35 years. These religious frameworks were identified for their doctrines and teachings or their involvement with legal proceedings for child neglect. Not all religions have had children become gravely ill or die due to prayer in lieu of medical care, nor do all church members follow the doctrines or teachings of particular religions that promote withholding medical care for their members. The purpose of the latter part of Chapter 4 is to present information from the literature, media, or interviews about religions that have been identified as having doctrines that *influence* healthcare decisions for children. The intent is not to judge or make accusations. Rather, the intent is to inform healthcare professionals about identified religions or churches whose doctrines have *potential* to influence medical healthcare decisions.

Some churches embraced investigation; others would not return phone calls or letters of inquiry. Still others could not be located and were identified solely on the basis of legal or media summaries covering examples of treatment refusal.

# CHURCHES WITH FRAMEWORKS SUPPORTING REFUSAL OF MEDICAL TREATMENT OR REFUSAL

The following list includes 31 religious groups found in the current literature whose doctrines or teachings have been noted to influence decisions about children's healthcare:

1) Jehovah's Witnesses

2) Christian Science

3) The Church of the First Born

4) Christian Catholic Church (Not affiliated with the Roman Catholic Church)

5) Faith Assembly

6) Followers of Christ

7) End Time Ministries

8) The Believers' Fellowship

9) Faith Temple Doctoral Church of Christ in God

10) The Source

11) Christ Miracle Healing Center

12) "No Name" Fellowship

13) The Fellowship

14) Faith Tabernacle Congregation

15) 1st Century Gospel

16) Pentecostal Church

17) Evangelistic Healers

18) Jesus Through Jon and Judy

19) Wiccans (people who identify themselves as Witches; not a religious order)

20) Four Square Church

21) Christ Assembly

22) The Church of God of the Union Assembly

23) Church of God Chapel

24) Northeast Kingdom Community Church

25) True Followers of Christ

26) Faith Cathedral Assembly

27) Living Word Assembly of God

28) Traveling Ministries Everyday Church

29) Bible Readers Fellowship

30) The Body (a.k.a. The Body of Christ)

31) Oregon-based Christ Church

(Asser & Swan, 1998; CHILD, n.d.; Massachusetts Citizens for Children, n.d.; Ontario Consultants on Religious Tolerance, n.d.; Swan, 1997; Swan, 2000).

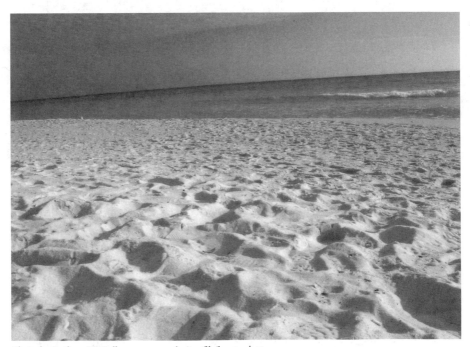

*Photo by Kathryn McCallum. www.sxc.hu/profile/lemon-drop*

Kostinchuk (2001) offers brief examples of a number of the above religions. In his descriptions of their beliefs, he sheds light on how they receive public awareness. He titles them the "players" and offers this information with numerous helpful references:

1) The Bible Readers Fellowship, an evangelical group located in California, does not report or record births or deaths as required by state law. The group supports avoidance of all medical treatments.

2) Members of the End Time Ministries sect hold faith healing as a high belief. They reject medical interventions for their children and do not allow healthcare professionals to be present at the births of their babies.

3) Members of the Oregon-based Christ Church believe in the power of prayer as a cure for medical conditions. They prefer to use anointing oils and "laying on of hands" rather than traditional medical interventions, even for their children.

4) Many Pentecostal sects also believe in "laying on of hands" rather than seeking medical attention for their members (including children).

5) Faith Tabernacle Congregation Church members believe they can be cured of sickness by the prayers of "true believers." Members who seek medical care are seen by some members as turning their backs on God and their faith.

6) According to followers of the General Assembly Church of The First Born, the sovereign power of God to heal is the center of their belief system.

7) Members of the Faith Tabernacle Church are encouraged to follow what the group sees as God's will, including the notion that God's will is to not seek medical treatment, even for church members' children.

*Keep in mind that many people within religions believe in prayer and supernatural healing as a possibility.*

Unfortunately, most of the 31 religious groups listed on the previous pages do not have accessible information about the particulars of their religious doctrines. When a healthcare professional encounters a "family of faith" about whom there is little knowledge, the best source of information is the family itself. With great respect for privacy, the professional healthcare provider should ask probing questions to assess the family's individualized interpretation of the belief system, using a tone of acceptance. If fear arises, the opportunity for subsequent conversations or precious negotiations may be lost. Keep in mind that many people within religions believe in prayer and supernatural healing as a possibility. For the majority of people, medical care is readily accepted along with spiritual practices.

# TYPES OF PRAYER AND RELIGIOSITY INFLUENCING HEALTHCARE DECISIONS

*With the sudden explosion of nontraditional healing practices and the use of integrated, holistic, and alternative health treatments, there has been a great deal of attention given to the influence of religion, prayer, and consciousness on treatment decisions and health outcomes.*

The study of the influence of religiosity on healthcare decisions dates back to the 19th century and is found in more than 250 published empirical studies. Few of the studies published were explicitly designed to investigate religion. Rather, most were intended to identify the relationship of health outcomes, morbidity, and mortality to one or more religious indicators.

According to Levin (1994), healthcare professionals have not historically recognized that religious backgrounds are influential to healthcare decisions. "As a result, the idea that one's religious background or experiences might in some way influence one's health has remained part of the folklore of discussion on the fringes of the research community" (p. 1475). Times have changed. With the sudden explosion of nontraditional healing practices and the use of integrated, holistic, and alternative health treatments, there has been a great deal of attention given to the influence of religion, prayer, and consciousness on treatment decisions and health outcomes. The Institute of Noetic Sciences, located in Northern California, is currently conducting empirical research on the power of prayer (also called intention by Noetic members) in healing, including experiments on the results of local and distant prayer (intention) on physiological measurements (Issues on Spirituality and Research Lecture Series, 2001).

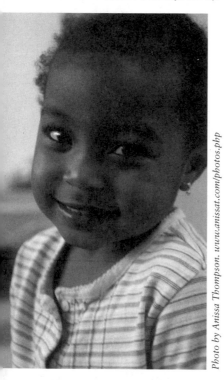

Photo by Anissa Thompson. www.anissat.com/photos.php

Dr. Jeffery S. Levin, MPH, a former medical school professor and epidemiologist, has published numerous articles and several books that support the link between prayer and health. His articles review evidence found within hundreds of epidemiologic studies that have reported statistically significant findings (which he calls salutary effects) between religious indicators on reported morbidity and mortality. His research has led to the development of further questions, including "Is it valid?" and "Is it causal?" His research has led to evidence that says "yes," "probably," and "maybe" (Levin, 1994). Levine has continued to study the connection between faith and healing and has published five books, several based on international research, on the areas of the relationship among faith, healing, and prayer. According to Levine's personal Web site, http://www.religionandhealth.com/abstracts90s.html, questions still posed include: 1) What is the transcendence experience? 2) What is the role of faith, spirituality, and healing? 3) Can the transcendence experience be studied? 4) How can religious faith serve as a resource for the prevention of illness and the promotion of well-being? A final causal summation remains difficult.

Levin's (1994) extensive review of hundreds of published research articles on the relationship of religiosity and health identified many confounding variables, including:

1) strict lifestyle or health-related behaviors sanctioned by religious denominations;

2) heredity as morbidity and mortality in particular groups of shared religious beliefs (Tay-Sachs in Ashkenazi Jews, sickle cell anemia in blacks, and hypercholesterolemia in Dutch Reformed Afrikaners);

3) psychosocial effects, since many religious denominations provide intense social support, possibly buffering anger and stress;

4) psychodynamics of belief systems, which may engender purpose, peacefulness, and self-confidence (or the alternative); and

5) psychodynamics of faith or the mere belief that religious beliefs of God are health-enhancing, which may be enough to produce salutary effects.

One example in Levin's (1994) article is the lower incidence of hypertension found in several religious groups. Seventh-day Adventists are noted to be healthier than members of other religious groups, especially in regard to hypertension. This may be attributed to their shared doctrine of not eating meat; an emphasis on family solidarity, religious fellowship and self-responsibility; and their encouragement of self-care and beneficial health-related behaviors. Levin suggests that there is a religion-health association, which may be valid, but a comprehensive meta-analysis to disclose ample empirical associations does not currently exist.

In general, the study of prayer as a healing tool poses problems and challenges for both the court systems, which have the responsibility to distinguish the validity of prayer as an alternative for medical care, and for researchers, who are seeking to validate prayer through such means as clinical trials. According to Dusek, Astin, Hibberd, and Krucoff (2003), there is an absence of knowledge and tangible evidence, or even the mechanism of a healing energy (or force), with prayer. These authors describe how the conduction of prospective randomized controlled clinical trials may not be necessary if the primary objective of a research study is to discover the philosophical underpinnings. According to the authors, the application of clinical trial designs possesses the risk of being overly reductionistic and detrimental. They offer two central assumptions:

1) Therapy studies must be sufficiently definable to be integrated into healthcare systems, facilitated as a human resource of wellness or recovery, or manipulated as a therapy applied professionally.

2) Therapeutic impact on the combined mind-body-spirit continuum must include some measurable somatic component (Dusek et al., 2003, p. A44).

The research on prayer efficacy remains wide open. Some researchers have used high-quality methods and others have not. Some of the reports using high-quality clinical trials have demonstrated prayer as a positive treatment, while others show no effect of prayer on healing. No clear patterns have emerged demonstrating which clinical conditions are most responsive to the effects of prayer, as most research has been conducted with considerable heterogeneity of diseases (Dusek et al., 2003).

One needs to ask if prayer can indeed be scientifically studied as an actual healthcare intervention. With this question in mind, three distinct problems (among others) have emerged in the study of prayer:

1) the theological concerns that prayer studies attempt to manipulate God or reduce Divine influence to equations seeking causal relationships;

2) the scientific concern over the absence of plausible or known mechanisms for which healing prayer might actually influence health; and

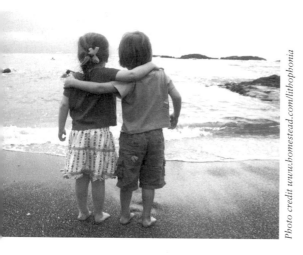

*Photo credit www.homestead.com/lithophonia*

3) the concerns over the definition of "dose of prayer" and the concerns over the manner in which the prayer is provided (Dusek et al., 2003).

There have been no concrete suggestions put forth in the current literature to guide researchers through these problems. Research continues to be conducted with a milieu of interventional mechanisms.

# CLERICAL INTERPRETATIONS

Prayer itself has been defined in many ways. The following section is devoted to definitions of various types of prayer, including clerical definitions, how the prayer is constructed, and how the prayer might be offered.

## PRAYER AS AN ALTERNATIVE OR COMPLEMENTARY THERAPY

Prayer has been considered as an alternative or an adjunct to traditional Western medical care for decades. Only recently has prayer become a focus of empirical study. People of diverse cultures and associations have used prayer as an alternative or in conjunction with treatments with tremendously successful testimonies. Prayer can be distant or near (at the bedside). It can be individualized or offered in groups.

According to Dr. Michael Lerner, president of Commonweal and co-creator of the Commonweal Cancer Help Program in Bolinas, CA, prayer has been studied as an adjunct to traditional Western medical care to identify its therapeutic effects. In *Choices in Healing: Integrating the Best of Conventional and Complementary Approaches to Cancer* (1994), Lerner describes the outcome of a study performed by Dr. Randolph Byrd at San Francisco General Medical Center. Byrd's research was designed to determine whether intercessory prayer (prayer for a patient by others) offered by born-again Christians, as described by the Gospel of John 3:3, offered a therapeutic effect in conjunction with traditional prayer. The study found six conditions were improved. These conditions were:

1) the need for intubation or ventilation

2) the need for antibiotics

3) the incidence of cardiopulmonary arrest

4) the incidence of congestive heart failure

5) the incidence of pneumonia

6) the need for diuretics

The study group ($n = 393$, 192 in the intervention group and 201 in the control group) demonstrated a general tendency for better physical outcomes than did the control group, who were not prayed for (Lerner, 1994).

## INTERCESSORY PRAYER

Dr. Dwight Conrad (personal communication, April 23, 2005), whose ministerial career has spanned both theological study and pastoral care, defined intercessory prayer in the following essay:

> A fundamental moral fact of Creation is the *freedom of will and of choice*. Nothing—no one—countermands that law. Even Jesus, having prophesied Peter's denial, could do nothing for His friend except surround him with the atmosphere of caring love: "But I have prayer for you Peter" (Luke 22:32).
>
> The *Basic Act of Intercession* is a caring love that establishes a spiritual climate around the objects of our prayers, within which consent to change is possible. So Jesus prays (in His Great Prayer, John 17:15-20), "I pray not that they be taken out of the world ... but that in their situations they may be protected." Secondly, intercession asks that the intercessor identify with the object with his or her prayers. Moses, after the golden calf fiasco, pleads with God, "Do not destroy this people in Your anger; but, if you must slay them, slay me as well" (Exodus 32:32; Numbers 14:1-20). In Genesis 18:16-35, Abraham argues with God for the souls of the people living in Sodom and Gomorrah.
>
> Thirdly, intercession demands *association* with the sinner. So Jesus ate with (was accused of eating with) the dregs of society: publicans and sinners (Matthew 9:11). Likewise, when Moses' sister, Miriam, was to be punished with leprosy for rebelling against him and against God, Moses not only prayed for her but accompanied her to her confinement outside the camp until she could be pronounced "clean" (Numbers 13:1-15).
>
> Fourthly, intercessory prayer requires *constancy and depth*. In Deuteronomy 9:26, Moses says, "For forty days and for forty nights I have lain prostrate before the Lord because of your sin." St. James, in his Epistle, reminds us, "The effectual, fervent prayer of a righteous man availeth much"

(James 5:16 in the King James Version; New International Version: "The constant prayer of a righteous man is effective and powerful."). An additional byword of intercessory prayer is *caring love* (agape and charitas in Greek). In John's Gospel (3:16), we are reminded, "For God so loved (agape) the world that He gave His only begotten Son so that whoever chooses to believe in Him shall not perish but shall have everlasting life." Job, even after the accusations and recriminations of his "friends" (Eliphaz, Bildad, and Zophar) continually prayed for them (Job 42:9).

## PRAYER IN ACTION

*The distance prayer operated on two principles: the basic contract of the intention to pray and the released energy posited by the suggestion of that prayer.*

Conrad continues to describe how those who apply prayer do so with suggestion and intention. He describes how the goal of distance intervention (intercessory prayer) is to effect wholeness in another person who is the object of that prayer. According to Conrad, because of human freedom, we are in actuality praying for a Divine atmosphere of healing energy to surround the prayer object. The "object" must accept this atmosphere of healing energy for the prayer to be effective. Conrad continues to say that for this reason, it is essential that those for whom the prayer is offered are aware that such prayer is being offered.

Several studies suggest that this "knowledge" is most advantageous in releasing individual healing potential. One researcher reports that a client asked her to pray for him at a specific hour on a subsequent day during which he would undergo a difficult medical procedure. The re-

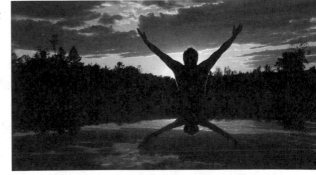

*Photo by Bill Davenport. www.lightshadow.blogspot.com*

searcher, busy with other clients and demands on her time, forgot the promised prayer appointment. Realizing her mistake, she went to the patient's room to apologize for her behavior. She found, contrary to her expectations, a welcoming smile from the patient, who reported (and the doctors verified) distinct and instantaneous physical improvement at that moment when the patient believed that the requested prayer had been offered for him (D. Conrad, personal communication, May 23, 2005). Conrad states that in this case, the distance prayer operated on two principles: the basic contract of the *intention* to pray and the released energy posited by the *suggestion* of that prayer. The model for this kind of prayer is found in the New Testament in the Gospel of St. John, Chapter 17, commonly called "The Great High Priestly Prayer of Jesus." The outline of the prayer is simple:

1) Jesus is specific;

2) he is empathetic;

3) he prays for Divine influence for His disciples but not for the abrogation of their freedom;

4) he offers thanksgiving that His prayer has been heard;

5) he "suggests" to His disciples the content of His prayer.

*Those patients for whom prayer was intended were five times less likely than the control patients to require antibiotics and three times less likely to develop pulmonary edema.*

A study of intercessory prayer efficacy was conducted by cardiologist Randolph Byrd, MD, and published in 1998 in the peer-reviewed *Southern Medical Journal*. He used a randomized, double-blind protocol to study the possible effects of intercessory prayer in a sample of coronary care unit (CCU) patients. Over 10 months, 393 patients admitted to the CCU were, with informed consent, randomly placed in either a prayer group (192) or in a control group (201). Prayer was provided by devout intercessors outside of the hospital. Neither patients nor the evaluating physicians were aware of which people were designated to receive prayers. It was found that, although these individuals were well-matched at their hospital entry, the prayed-for patients showed significantly superior recovery compared to those for whom no prayer was offered. Those patients for whom prayer was intended were five times less likely than the control patients to require antibiotics and three times less likely to develop pulmonary edema. None of the patients in the prayer group required endotracheal intubation, whereas 12 patients in the control group required mechanical ventilation support. Fewer prayed-for patients than control-group patients died. The difference in this area of the study, while individually satisfactory, is not statistically significant. The design and the results of the Byrd study are impressive, and even skeptical commentators seem to agree on the significance of his findings.

## FAITH HEALING

Religious affiliations promoting faith-healing measures to the exclusion of medical care are not new. Faith healing has been well-documented for more than 200 years. An example of a faith-healing sect is the General Assembly Church of the First Born, whose members consider it a sin to seek medical care above God's power to heal. Amanda Bates, whose parents were part of the General Assembly Church of the First Born in Colorado, died of complications of untreated diabetes while her parents prayed over her (Dyer, 2000). Another example of an application of faith healing concerns a religious group-healing procedure given to an adolescent who complained of a migraine headache. The group of faithful adults circled the child and described to her that her headaches were not real; rather, they were the result of sinful behaviors and sinful thoughts. The leader of the group continued to "praise God for His amazing power of healing" and "shunned the devil for causing

pain and disease in the natural world." The child was instructed to ask for forgiveness, keeping her eyes closed while the group "laid on" healing hands. At the conclusion of the prayer session, the girl remained calm, eyes closed for a long period of time, and reported that the headache was resolving. They kept her in bed for an hour or more after the healing session (H. Conrad, personal communication, May 24, 2005).

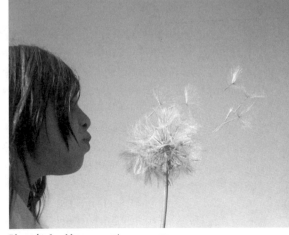

*Photo by Jyn Meyer. www.jynmeyer.com*

Faith healings can take place in dyads, small or large groups, and staged gatherings. Sometimes cults or religious groups will charge an entry fee for attending faith-healing sessions. The one being healed may pay more for the cure.

## DIVINE HEALING

The term *divine healing* is used by church organizations such as Seventh-day Adventists. The term itself has many meanings for many different groups of people. Conrad writes:

> Prayer presupposes that there is an intimate connection between the Creator and the Creation. Every theological system, every religion, posits this "connectedness." In primitive societies, it was believed that everything we use, all that we touch, and the "unseen" beyond the sensory, is populated by spirits similar to ours (in some sense) to which we can relate and which may intimately affect our lives—these beliefs all fall under the general heading of animism. Our more sophisticated theologies attempt to reconcile the divine/human international continuum by theorizing several ways this interaction may be facilitated:
>
> 1)   Through creational and evolutionary similarities between that which creates and that which is created. In the Judeo-Christian tradition, the Creation Myth of Genesis solves this problem as God "creates man in His own image" (Genesis 1:26).
>
> 2)   Through the dual nature of divine/human entities (God-men), this interconnectedness may be understood and accomplished: Within the Christian tradition, this is the doctrine of the Incarnation within which Jesus is both God and man, the Second Person of the Trinity. Hebrews 4:15 enunciates the doctrinal basis for this connection, "For we have not a High Priest who is unable to sympathize with our weaknesses; but we have One who was tempted in all points *just as we are.*" Egyptian, Roman, and Greek pantheons all contain similar divine/human personages whose function is to foster identification, understanding, and connection.

3)  Through especially gifted interpreters such as prophets in the Old Testament in Judaism, bodhisattvas in Buddhism, mediums and spirit guides in modern psychicism, the "familiars" of Wicca and covens, and "healers" in Christian Science and similar systems.

Prayer presupposes it is both possible and desirable for humans to address the Divine. It is understandable that an omnipotent Deity might speak to its creation, but for prayer to be operative we must believe, if only arrogantly so, that that which is created may also speak to the creator. And yet another prayer presupposes that the Divine is both capable of response and disposed to respond. In the Old Testament, God is called, "You who answer prayer" (Psalms 65:2; 1 Kings 9:3). This understanding of God is reflected in the New Testament in the Gospel of St. Matthew 7:11. Behind all praying that eventuates healing is this presupposition that God is kindly disposed to intervene in human affairs for our benefit. Two caveats are necessary here: Our intention in prayer is not the reformation of God's will and purpose but the conformation of our energies and attentions with God's toward an identified purpose; benefits cover a wide range of Divine prayer response, from the reinterpretations of our situations (pain, for instance, may not necessarily be eliminated, but the mind's obsessions and fears may, through prayer, be refocused and more easily borne) to actual healing and well-being. (D. Conrad, personal communication, 2005)

Prayer is a complex human interest that can be viewed through many different lenses. Prayer used for healing has a special lens, since those who participate have a particular goal—to call upon external forces to provide care, healing, support, comfort, direction, and evidence of presence and relationship.

*Behind all praying that eventuates healing is this presupposition that God is kindly disposed to intervene in human affairs for our benefit.*

# Specific Religious Doctrines Defined

Of the 31 previously listed religions with doctrines that reference to parents' healthcare decisions for their children, not all can be substantiated or validated through reputable sources. Therefore, the following section includes descriptions only for the most prevalent doctrines that are verifiable via reputable sources in the literature.

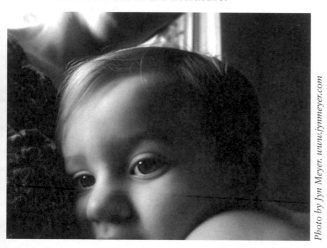

*Photo by Jyn Meyer. www.jynmeyer.com*

It is important to reinforce the point that not all church members follow religious doctrines. Nor do all individual churches affiliated with the 31 religions listed earlier in this chapter teach the doctrines, faith-healing practices, or prayer sessions that may influence healthcare decisions that could ultimately endanger children's lives. Individual congregational members may adopt behaviors, beliefs, and values based on their own interpretations of biblical passages, or they may follow the lead of strict or radical church members or leaders who are highly influential regarding the adherence of religious teachings and healthcare decisions.

The first two religious doctrines that will be described come from the Jehovah's Witnesses Church and the Christian Science Church. These churches are reputable institutions with a worldwide membership base, and both have doctrines that highly influence treatment decisions. Following these presentations, an evangelical church will be briefly described. The selection of the churches to be discussed was based solely on the amount of legitimate and reputable sources of literature found.

## Jehovah's Witnesses

In the 1870s, the foundations of the Jehovah's Witnesses (JW) sect were built as a nondenominational study group by Charles Taze Russell (1852-1916), a Pennsylvanian. By 1909, this first study group had spawned study groups all over the world that focused on biblical prophecy, and the Watchtower

Bible and Tract Society—the official name of the JW organization—became international. In 1927, the first biblical publication was disseminated forbidding blood transfusion on penalty of loss of eternal life in God's kingdom (Vercillo & Duprey, 1988). JW have interpreted the most frequently cited verses of the Bible as making references that:

> Every moving thing that lives shall be food for you ... only you shall not eat flesh with its life, that is, its blood. (Genesis 8:3-4)

> For it has seemed good to the Holy Spirit and to us to lay upon you ... these necessary things: that you abstain from what has been sacrificed to idols and from blood. (Acts 15:28-29).

> You must not eat the blood of any sort of flesh, because the soul of every sort of flesh is its blood. Anyone eating it will be cut off. (Leviticus 17:13-14; Thurkauf, 1989, p. 119-204)

Denouncement of blood transfusions by the Watchtower Society took place in the 1940s. According to Swan (1997), the timing was curious in that during that time period, Witnesses were refusing to sing the national anthem. Swan, describes how the 1940s' media coverage emphasized that donating blood was a patriotic duty. Some consider the two to be related.

The underlying theme to JW teachings is the consequences of disobedience. According to Quintero (1993), the church's belief system states:

> If God's directive is not obeyed, eternal life is forfeited. If they disobey God and are "cut-off," believers will be denied life through resurrection. If a person's life is extended by a transfusion, it will become meaningless and lack spiritual purpose because the hope of everlasting life has been forfeited. (p. 46)

As described by Quintero's (1993) article on blood administration in pediatrics, JW believe that violation means loss of salvation, and some insist that the negative spiritual effects are incurred regardless of whether the person actually chooses the blood transfusion. Other JW disagree and assert that if the recipient is unconscious, or blood is transfused against the patient's will, the soul is not affected.

The challenge for healthcare professionals is not that JW genuinely believe they have responsibility for their child's food, shelter, and healthcare (Quintero, 1993), but that their faith will allow their own child's death before they would go against their interpretation of the Bible and consent for transfusion (Vercillo & Duprey, 1988). They will defend their right to make medical decisions for their children on the basis that, as parents, they are responsible adults (Quintero, 1993).

With all the pharmaceutical and technological progress we encounter daily in the healthcare arena, there are still very few alternatives to blood transfusions. (See Table 1 for a summary of the latest technology in this area.) Based on literature reports, conflicts exist within the JW community, as some adherents will accept blood-based treatments but not blood itself (Muramoto, 1999). (See Table 2 for a list of components and procedures acceptable or unacceptable within the JW faith, compiled by Watchtower Society publications and from statements by JW physicians. See Table 3 for a list of generally accepted treatment options and procedures.)

*They will defend their right to make medical decisions for their children on the basis that, as parents, they are responsible adults*

### Table 1

**LATEST TECHNOLOGY IN ALTERNATIVES FOR BLOOD TRANSFUSIONS**

Maximize blood production:
> Erythropoietin
> Intravenous iron dextran
> Nutritional support, including calories and amino acids for red blood cell production

Maximize cardiac output:
> Volume expansion via synthetic colloids and crystalloid solutions such as:
>> Hydroxyethyl starch (HES)
>> Dextran 40 and Dextran 70
>> Urea-bridged gelatin
>> Modified fluid gelatin
> Hemodilution

Increase oxygen content:
> Oxygen
> Fluorinated blood substitutes that carry oxygen

Decrease metabolic rate:
> Hypothermia (targeting core temperatures of 30-32 degrees Celsius to reduce oxygen consumption by 40%)
> Paralysis with ventilatory support to prevent oxygen-consuming shivering
> Sedation

Minimize blood losses:
> Microchemistry analyzers
> Pediatric-sized blood samples
> Sterile reservoirs
> Hypotensive anesthesia in intra-operative procedures
> Desmopressin to reduce blood loss after cardiopulmonary bypass surgery

Surgical procedures:
> Hypotensive anesthesia
> Local infiltration with vasopressors
> Preliminary ligation of major arteries

Yet to be developed:
> Genetically engineered pig hemoglobin solutions
> Human hemoglobin solutions
> Longer half-life solutions of fluorocarbon preparations

Habler, O. (2005). Blood safety: Artificial oxygen carriers offer an alternative to red blood cell transfusion. Obesity, Fitness & Wellness Week. 3 December 2005. Retrieved 21 August 2006 from: http://www.newsrx.com/newsletters/Obesity,-Fitness-and-Wellness-Week/2005-12-03/1203200533396OW.html

Spahn, D.R., Kocian, R. (2005). Artificial oxygen carriers: Status in 2005. Current Pharmaceutical Design. 2005;11(31):4099-114.

Stubbs, J.R. (2006). Alternatives to blood transfusion in critically ill: Erythropoietin. Critical Care Medicine. May; 34 (5 Supplement). 5106-0.

Sung, K.C., et al. (2006). In pediatric cardiac surgery, hydroxyethyl starch is a safe alternative for volume replacement. Obesity, Fitness & Wellness Week. 25 March 2006. Retrieved 21 August 2006 from http://www.newsrx.com/newsletters/Obesity,-Fitness-and-Wellness-Week/2006-03-25/0325200633315240OW.html

*Table 2*

## PROCEDURES ACCEPTABLE OR UNACCEPTABLE TO JEHOVAH'S WITNESSES

Whole Blood
> Unacceptable if taken as "blood transfusion"
> Acceptable if taken as contained in bone marrow transplant

Plasma proteins
> Unacceptable if taken as "plasma"
> Acceptable if taken separately as individual blood components such as albumin, clotting factors, or fibrin

White Blood Cell Transfusion
> Unacceptable if taken as "white blood cell transfusion"
> Acceptable if taken as "peripheral stem cell transfusion"

Autologous Blood
> Unacceptable if tube connection to the patient's body is interrupted
> Acceptable if the tube to the body is maintained, such as hemodilution or a cell-saver machine to capture and re-infuse one's blood during or after surgical procedures

Stem Cell Transfusion
> Unacceptable if taken from umbilical cord blood
> Acceptable if taken from peripheral circulation or bone marrow

Heart-Lung Machine Technology
> Unacceptable if patient's blood is used to prime the machine
> Acceptable if the patient's blood is used to circulate the machine after priming

Epidural Blood Patch
> Unacceptable if blood is removed from the vein and injected back into the patient
> Acceptable if the blood is injected through a syringe that is connected to the vein via a continuous tube system

Blood Donations

Unacceptable if the blood is donated by Jehovah's Witnesses for use of other Jehovah's Witnesses and others

Acceptable if donated by non-Jehovah's Witness for use of Jehovah's Witness and others (and only for use of blood components, not as packed cell transfusion, whole blood transfusion, or other intact blood in its non-single component form)

*(Muramoto, 1999, p. 298)*

## Table 3

### STATUS OF ACCEPTABILITY OF PROCEDURES FOR JEHOVAH'S WITNESSES

Generally Accepted:

**Crystalloid intravenous solutions** (for blood volume expansion)

Ringer's Lactate

Normal saline solutions

Hypertonic saline solutions

**Colloids** (used to replace lost plasma proteins)

Dextran

Gelatin

Hetastarch

**Perfluorochemicals** (chemicals used in the lungs to increase oxygen/carbon dioxide exchange)

**Erythropoietin** (medication used to promote the production of red blood cells from the bone marrow)

Generally Not Accepted:

**Whole blood transfusions** (often used during emergencies to quickly restore blood volume)

**Packed red blood cell transfusions** (most frequently used form of transfusion therapy)

*continues*

*Table 3* *continued*

## STATUS OF ACCEPTABILITY OF PROCEDURES FOR JEHOVAH'S WITNESSES

**Leukocyte transfusions** (used in extreme states of neutropenia to boost the immune system)

> **Plasma** (used for clotting factors and infrequently used for blood volume expansion)

> **Auto-transfusions** (used when one's condition allows the collection and banking of one's own blood for later use, thus reducing the chances of being exposed to the foreign proteins or possible infectious diseases that one can be exposed to during donated blood transfusions)

Left up to Individual Decisions

> **Cardiopulmonary bypass technology** (used for cardiac and pulmonary emergencies and surgeries)

> **Dialysis** (used to correct conditions such as renal failure—removes the accumulation of human waste products circulating in the blood)

> **Plasmapheresis** (a process technology used to divide blood components for separate infusion)

> **Immune globins** (used as a mechanism of passive immunity against certain infectious diseases)

> **Vaccines** (used as a form of passive immunity for the prevention of infectious diseases)

> **Sera** (used as a serum replacement for volume expansion)

> **Hemophilia preparations** (used when a genetic condition leads to the absence of one of a number of clotting factors, now via recombinant technology—no longer taken from pooled blood)

> **Transplants** (can be tissue or organs)

*(Mann, Votto, Kambe, & McNamee, 1992, p. 1043)*

The conflict surrounding freedom of choice for JW has been presented in the current literature by Muramoto (1999). He reports that the Watchtower Society does not give church members the freedom to accept blood therapy without penalty. According to Muramoto, JW who accept a blood-based product and do not repent of the action before a judicial committee will receive the harshest sanction of the religion—disfellowship or excommunication. Because accepting transfusions is considered betraying God, the offender will be socially isolated and shunned by church members.

In contrast, Heller (1998) reports JW church members do not censure members who choose to take another course (seeking transfusions). He quotes James Pellechia, director of public affairs for JW, as saying: "We believe in seeking the best medical help for ourselves and our families. It is the Christian thing to do. If someone caves under pressure, we offer aid and support, do what we can pastorally to help the family" (p. 2).

When dealing with blood transfusion situations involving JW, it is critical for the healthcare team to demonstrate that the blood transfusion (or blood product) is lifesaving. Courts have been known to refuse a petition for an order for JW children with sickle cell disease and JW children who need preoperative or intraoperative transfusions (Quintero, 1993). Yet, according to Tierney, Weinberger, Greene, and Studdard (1984), "To date, there has been no case in which medical personnel have been refused temporary guardianship when the child's life was clearly in danger" (p. 477).

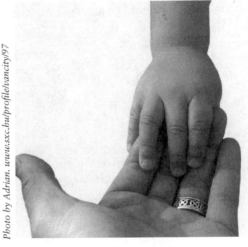

Photo by Adrian. www.sxc.hu/profile/vancity/97

Many JW seek "contracts" from their physicians that no blood products will be transfused under any conditions. Alternatively, church members have been known to sign a statement agreeing to absolve the physician and healthcare team from all responsibility. In dealing with the immediate healthcare needs of children during life-or-death decision-making situations, physicians might not accept these statements and instead may continue to petition to the courts for temporary legal guardianship so that transfusion therapy can be used. According to Migden and Braen (1998), it is general practice that adult JW carry with them a card that speaks to their desire to refuse blood, even if deemed lifesaving by the attending physician.

In 1998, there were more than 3.2 million Jehovah's Witnesses worldwide, of which 25% resided in the United States. In 2002, there were more than 6 million worldwide, with 1 million in the United States and 100,000 in Canada, including hundreds of healthcare professionals, surgeons, and physicians (Bodnaruk, Wong & Thomas, 2004).

What these statistics reinforce is that healthcare professionals must be fully aware of the need to meticulously assess the situation and deem treatments *lifesaving* before petitioning courts for temporary guardianship. All alternatives to blood transfusion and all alternatives to those treatments considered unacceptable to the religion must be considered prior to transfusion. Whenever possible, in emergency and nonemergency situations, clergy and family members should be consulted prior to proceeding with standard transfusion therapy.

*Healthcare professionals must be fully aware of the need to meticulously assess the situation and deem treatments lifesaving before petitioning courts for temporary guardianship.*

There is now a group within the greater JW membership that is pushing to reform the position on transfusion therapy. The group, known as the Associated Jehovah's Witnesses for Reform on Blood (or AJWRB), uses a Web site as its primary mode of communication for discussing and advocating for reform of the church's blood stance. This group advocates that, "A blood transfusion is a liquid tissue or organ transplant, not a meal, and hence does not violate the biblical admonition to abstain from (eating) blood" (Associated Jehovah's Witnesses for Reform on Blood, n.d.).

AJWRB, an international group representing members in many countries, calls for its members and other readers to be child advocates. The group encourages questioning those JW members who go door-to-door to explain how the Watchtower (the leadership base of JW) decides "which parts of blood God permits" (AJWRB, n.d.). The AJWRB calls for a termination of subsidizing the Watchtower Society's continued desire for legal exemptions, and the site requests that children's medical needs continue to be protected. The site also has a brief critique of a previously published *AWAKE!* magazine (published by the Watchtower Society) that featured 26 children who "put God first" and died because they did not receive blood transfusions. The AJWRB considers the loss of children's lives directly related to blood transfusion refusals to be first-degree murder.

JW has a strong international presence and seems to place significant value on the discussion of its beliefs—as witnessed firsthand by those who have been visited by Jehovah's Witnesses. According to Thurkauf (1989), Jehovah's Witnesses will be grateful if their beliefs are honored. The stress and anxiety of serious illness are still realities, and it is very important to continue to provide support in a nonjudgmental way. Tables 1-3 (see pages 68-72) provide a thorough overview of allowed and disallowed blood-based treatments. Knowledge of these policies can be very helpful to healthcare professionals faced with a blood transfusion refusal, as it will help the family feel more understood and less judged. Thus, this knowledge will help keep stress as low as possible during discussions and negotiations for necessary treatments. It is important to remember that for the family, making these decisions isn't easy, and supportive environments can go a long way toward easing the situation.

## CHRISTIAN SCIENTISTS

Mary Baker Eddy established the religious doctrine of the Church of Christ, Scientist—known mostly as Christian Science—in 1879. Church doctrines were based upon her own "divine" healing that occurred in 1866 after she read the New Testament's disclosure of Jesus' healing practices. In 1875, she wrote a book titled *Science and Health*, later published as *Science and Health with Key to the Scripture*. This text describes the principles of divine healing and laws expressed in the acts and sayings of Jesus. Christian Scientists teach that God is the only reality and that one can overcome sin, evil, and illness by understanding this principle. The teachings of Mary Baker Eddy clearly describe reliance on spiritual, rather than medical, means for healing. There are now Christian Science followers in 139 countries (The First Church of Christ, Scientist, n.d.), the greatest percentage being women, and although each church is self-governed and without individual pastors, two readers conduct each service with universally shared lessons, culled mainly from *Science and Health with Key to the Scripture.*

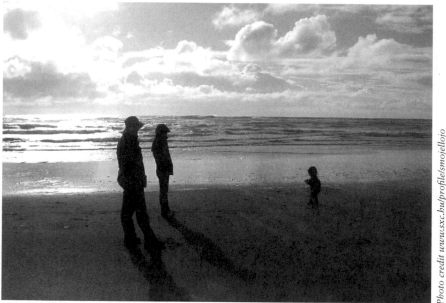

The numerous publications are the guiding communication of Christian Science beliefs. These publications include *The Christian Science Monitor*, *The Christian Science Quarterly Weekly Bible Lessons*, *The Herald of Christian Science*, *The Christian Science Sentinel*, and *The Christian Science Journal* (The First Church of Christ, Scientist, n.d.). The following six quotes from Mary Baker Eddy's 1875 book and 1925 teachings succinctly describe her doctrine:

> The prayer of faith shall save the sick, says the scripture. What is this healing prayer? A mere request that God will heal the sick has no power to gain more of the divine presence than is always at hand. The beneficial effect of such prayer for the sick is on the human mind, making it act more powerfully on the body through a blind faith in God. (Eddy, 1875, p. 12)

> The proof of truth, life and love, which Jesus gave by casting out error and healing the sick, completed his earthly mission; but in the Christian Church this demonstration of healing was early lost, about three centuries after philosophy, material medica, or scholastic theology ever taught or demonstrated the divine healing of absolute science. (Eddy, 1875, p. 41)

After a lengthy examination of my discovery and its demonstration in healing the sick, this fact became evident to me—that the mind governs the body, not partially but wholly. I submitted my metaphysical system of treating disease to the broadest practical tests. Since then, this system has gradually gained ground and has proved itself, whenever scientifically employed, to be the most effective curative agent in medical practice. (Eddy, 1875, p. 112)

Disease being a belief, a latent illusion of mortal mind, the sensation would not appear if the error of belief was met and destroyed by truth. If we understand the control of mind over body, we should put no faith in material means ... drugs and medicine. (Eddy, 1875, pp. 168-169)

A patient hears the doctor's verdict as a criminal hears his death sentence. The patient may seem calm under it, but he is not. His fortitude may sustain him, not his fear, which has already developed the disease that is gaining the mastery, is increased by the physician's words. (Eddy, 1875, p. 198)

Life in matter is a dream; sin, sickness and death are this dream. ... God made all that is made, but He never made sin or sickness. (Eddy, 1925)

A complex component to the Christian Scientist Church is its communications to its practitioners and "nurses," as they are to avoid administering any type of medicine or conduct behaviors that could be interpreted as practicing medicine. According to Swan (1997), the religion also has tenets that discourage the reporting of sick children who have had medical treatment refused or withheld, even though Christian Science practitioners are not exempt from state-mandated child abuse reporting for the withholding of medical treatment. Reporting suspected communicable diseases to health officials is also discouraged. This puts healthcare professionals at a disadvantage in treating children who have been identified as needing healthcare, yet it allows church members a chance to apply their scientific prayer in lieu of traditional medical care.

What happens when the prayer administered by faithful Christian Scientists does not work to cure disease? Swan (1997) reports that Christian Science "nurses" have attended to children who have died of meningitis, pneumonia, diabetes, and bowel obstructions. Reimbursement for Christian Science practitioners by third-party payers has been established in some states. A Blue Cross representative noted that, like psychiatric care, treatments by Christian Science practitioners is justified. Furthermore, Medicare, Medicaid, and many plans for government employees cover Christian Science practitioner treatments (Swan, 1997). The Internal Revenue Service also recognizes the charges of Christian Science nurses as deductible medical expenses (Swan, 1997).

Of interest are the state laws that allow Christian Science children exemptions in studying about diseases. The church claims that teaching children about disease and disease-related symptoms tends to undermine the teachings of the church's doctrine (Swan, 1997). Although the American Medical Association (AMA) has called for a removal of statutes giving religious exemptions from immunizations, no legislation has been passed to repeal them. Forty-eight states now have religious exemptions for immunizations. The Christian Science Church circulates lists of diseases that are required to be reported to health authorities and encourages its family members to follow the law and report them. In contradiction, the church does not describe the reportable diseases and claims that "ignorance of disease is desirable in healing it spiritually and warns against getting a medical diagnosis" (Swan, 1997, p. 500).

*In contradiction, the church does not describe the reportable diseases and claims that "ignorance of disease is desirable in healing it spiritually and warns against getting a medical diagnosis"*

The *New England Journal of Medicine* published a position paper in 1983 by the Christian Science Church. Several of the sentiments that relate to the church's beliefs and doctrines concerning children and healthcare were shared in this article, which is printed, in part, below.

> Christian Scientists are caring and responsible people who love their children and want only the best possible care for them. They would not have relied on Christian Science for healing—sometimes over four and even five generations in the same family—if this healing were only a myth. Yet they approach the subject of healing on the basis of a very different perspective from that of medical practice. (Talbot, 1983, p. 1641)

To them it is part of a whole religious way of life and is, in fact, the natural outcome of theology that underlies it. This theology, Christian Scientists believe, is both biblically based and deeply reasoned. Indeed, they speak of it as "scientific" because they believe its truth has been demonstrated through practical healing experience time and time again. Certainly, Christian Science is leagues apart from faith-healing groups that have aroused current concerns, and its adherents share neither the fundamentalist theology nor the rigidly proscriptive views of medicine characteristic of these groups. They are given neither to blind invoking of "miracles" nor passive submission to sickness as God's will. (Talbot, 1983, p. 1641)

If a patient decides to turn to medical care, the Christian Science practitioner—in the patient's own interests—releases the case in a supportive spirit and without reproach. And if a Christian Scientist decides on medical treatment, he or she should cooperate with the physician without entertaining mental reservations about the treatment, which, as many doctors might acknowledge, could be detrimental to its effectiveness. (Talbot, 1983, p. 1643)

Furthermore, members of this denomination take community concerns about the well-being of children with deep seriousness. They have a strong record of cooperation with pubic-health officials over the years. ... Christian Science parents would not object to the administration of on-the-spot first aid for their children. But in some instances they might prefer, after careful consideration, to have Christian Science treatment rather than hospitalization, surgery, or extended therapy. Again, however, prayer and reasoned judgment amid the exigencies of practical situations—rather than abstract criteria—tend to shape the choice of treatment in emergency situations. ... Christian Scientists also obey the law when vaccination is required (though requesting exemption when it is possible), and they have a physician or licensed midwife in attendance at childbirth. (Talbot, 1983, p. 1643)

The only purpose of Christian Scientists' work with legislators has been to ensure that the responsible use of prayer on behalf of children is not equated with abuse and neglect. Our society should consider very carefully just how far it is prepared to go in the direction of claiming to determine that the emphasis on spiritual healing in the New Testament must be held so suspect that it should be virtually proscribed by law. Christian Scientists believe that within the framework of existing law, states can adequately protect children without arbitrarily intruding on parental rights or abridging religious rights that are important to all. (Talbot, 1983, p. 1644)

There is no doubt that Christian Science parents love and care for their children. The adherence to the faithful perspective that disease does not exist, should not be named, and should not be treated with traditional medical care before prayer does influence the relationship among healthcare providers, public health officials, teachers, and families. The view that this is neglect or abuse must be looked at critically for each case encountered, and families should be supported in their care and concern for their children's welfare as well as their relationship with God. Healthcare professionals must balance parents' desires to pray for their child, bring in a Christian Science practitioner, and have the time to offer their services prior to instigating traditional treatment, but not at the expense of the child's wellness or life. Legislative battles continue concerning upholding medical exemptions for families of faith or concerning the proposed adoption of new exemption legislation; therefore, healthcare professionals of all disciplines must be aware of the religious tenets of this faith and be

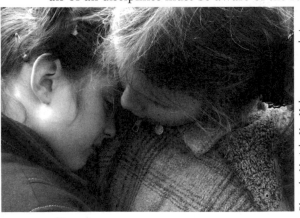

*Photo by Marinka Van Holten. www.sxc.hu/profile/Mrinkk*

prepared to act immediately on behalf of the child. The office of the nonprofit organization CHILD (Children's Healthcare Is a Legal Duty) contains case files of more than 30 deaths of Christian Science children between 1974 and 1994. These deaths were from ailments such as meningitis, pneumonia, septicemia, cancer, and measles. The strength of this church is remarkable, and continued study in the area of child health outcomes is warranted.

## FOLLOWERS OF CHRIST CHURCH

The Followers of Christ Church are a faithful group with wide representation. Mark Larabee (1998) reports how the Followers of Christ Church in Oregon City became notorious as having one of the largest faith-healing child mortality concentrations in the United States. A Followers of Christ Church member interviewed by Larabee describes a Christ- and Bible-stressing, tight-knit sect of Christian Bible-believers who encourage strict loyalty, an ardent faith in God and in divine healing, acceptance of the Lord's chastening as a parent's loving spanking, and suspicion of worldly outsiders. Members rely on the prayer closet (meetings of faithful members to apply faith-healing services directed by the pastor) and on faith-healing as Christ's channel of deliverance from evil of all kind.

It's not difficult to find Web-based biographical reports from former cult members who mourn the loss of their children. One such site—and note again that this site has not been verified for accuracy of the account—is www.geocities.com/Heartland/Woods/1327, which provides a critique of the death of a Followers of Christ member in 1983. According to this site, the group has a strong membership in northern and southern California, in addition to the Oregon City church. On this Web site, the author explains and mourns the loss of his 9-year-old daughter, Debbie, who died due to delayed medical care for a metastatic Wilms' (kidney) tumor. Debbie had been treated by the pastor with prayer and Bible-ordained intercession. The father described how they were faced with a dilemma when Debbie's condition worsened. He described their situation as being isolated and separatist, yet they decided to take Debbie to the child welfare authorities. After a brief hearing, the authorities initiated treatment for the child. One year later, after rigorous cancer treatment, Debbie died. The family was blamed by church members for not trusting God and leaving her life in His hands. The experience of Debbie's death caused shock for the parents. They felt the need to quit going to church and began to question the foundations of their faith.

> The poem of my heart was "Lord, I know you chasten your children, but chasten us, please don't take Debbie." Our grief was heavy. We were hurting and questioning. What good was all our "godly" zeal and intensity—if it couldn't

even save Debbie? What good was God, and what good were the doctors and all their optimism and the false-hopes they gave us?

It was hard for us to "let go and let God be God." But little by little we have gained peace. When she was dying, we were refreshed by so much kindness from those we did not expect it from. It was hard to comprehend that "outsiders" and un-believers, Samaritans, "lukewarm" believers and "worldly" doctors could have been so kind, while our own righteous zeal had stood judging them, closed (for so long) to their kindness. We found ourselves throwing out a lot of rules and enthusiasm, and turning to a much more basic and ordinary outlook. We came to see that God's healing is bigger than our private demands, that God is not just a God of this life, but surely the other one, too. That God is bigger than the narrow and exclusive sect we had formerly felt certain He had anointed as His special and select ones. When we were hurting and desperate, people of all kinds were trying to help, and it meant so much to us. It blessed us.

Indeed, even if there is truth in the scriptures which say we must not trust in man, we know God does use human inter-mediaries. (Shepherd, n.d., para. 11-13)

The above is an example of one family's experience with a path of faith crossed by an experience of doubt and loss attributable to that faith. Larabee (1998) reports that as of 1998, there were still 43 states that granted faith-healing parents sweeping immunities from prosecution on child neglect and abuse charges. Last updated in July 2005, CHILD, Inc.'s Web site reports that 48 states continue to have religious exemptions for particular healthcare provisions for children, while 39 states and the District of Columbia continue to have exemptions based on religious grounds for child abuse or neglect. CHILD, Inc. reports that 19 states continue to have religious exemptions to felony charges against parents, while 11 states continue to have exemptions against misdemeanors. Oregon is one of only six states that grant immunity on religious grounds for manslaughter, homicide or murder by abuse (Lara-bee, 1998).

*The people of the world can be seen as a tapestry woven of many different strands. Those strands differ in size, shape, color, intensity, age, and place of origin. All strands are integral to the whole, yet each retains an individuality that enriches the beauty of the cloth.*

5

# CULTURAL INFLUENCES TO TREATMENT REFUSAL

## OVERVIEW OF CULTURAL INFLUENCES

Race, ethnicity, and culture are three terms often misused in our healthcare system. The term *culture* is distinctly different, as a cultural group can represent several races and even ethnicities. According to Lipson, Dibble, and Minarik (1996), "The people of the world can be seen as a tapestry woven of many different strands. Those strands differ in size, shape, color, intensity, age, and place of origin. All strands are integral to the whole, yet each retains an individuality that enriches the beauty of the cloth" (p. iv). The cloth can be seen as cultural diversity, the strands as what each individual brings to the tapestry.

According to Lipson et al. (1996), "It is also important to understand and respect the healthcare culture within which the nurse is practicing. That culture, whether located within the hospital, home and/or community, is influenced by intersections of forces larger than the individual" (p. iv). Cultural norms are taught by many influencing factors. Individuals, such as cultural leaders, elders within a community, or even clergy, can be highly influential in creating cultural norms. Small groups within a larger cultural group also may influence what are considered to be acceptable behaviors or beliefs.

Similar to religious groups, not all members of every cultural group adopt the cultural norms that may influence parents' healthcare decisions for their children. Not all Muslims may subscribe to cultural norms pertaining to diet and lifestyle. Not all Jews aspire to religious norms required of faith-based Jewish members. Not all Hindus refuse beef-based medications and diets. Values seen within a cultural group may not be considered applicable to all group members. Autonomy, for example, may be highly valued by some members of a cultural group and not by others.

Several cultural groups have been found whose norms and cultural behaviors influence how parents make health-related decisions for their children. Examples of these cultural groups, found in recent literature and disclosed during ethnographic interviews with nurses and healthcare professionals, include Muslims, Hasidic Jews, Native American Indians, Hindus, Mexicans, and others. The following table represents examples of cultural practices or beliefs that may influence how parents make decisions for their children who enter the healthcare arena.

*Table 5*

| Examples of Cultural Influences to Healthcare Decisions for Children |
| --- |

Black Muslims:
> 1) Vegan diets.
> 2) Refusal of pork-based medicine.

Islamic Muslims:
> 1) May refuse narcotics or any medicines for children deemed addictive or with an alcohol base.
> 2) May refuse physical exams for their female children conducted by male healthcare providers.
> 3) May refuse pork foods and pork-based medicine, as it is seen as forbidden by God.

Hindus:
> 1) Refusal of beef-based medical products.
> 2) May need time for cultural pratices before consenting to treatment, surgeries, or diagnostics.

Haitians
   1) Supernatural illnesses may orginate from angry voodoo spirits, enemies, or the dead.
   2) Natural illnesses orginate from naural causes such as hot/cold or changes in blood flow, viscosity, purity, or temperature.

Native American Indians:
   1) May seek tribal leadership to approve chemo treatments or some surgeries for tribal children.
   2) Members who practice traditional medicine, which does not recognize "silent disease," may be reluctant to accept or participate in routine screening (Lipson et al., 1996).
   3) Cause of illness may be related to a violation of a prohibition or a restriction.
   4) Medicine and theology are strongly related.
   5) Singers may cure with their song; other specialists may use herbs; medical healers may use rituals.

Arabs:
   1) May refuse early ambulation after child's surgery to conserve energy for healing.

Chinese:
   1) May use acupuncturist or herbal medicine specialists prior to seeking modern interventions.
   2) Very modest and polite.
   3) Superstitious.

Vietnamese:
   1) Parents may not wish children to become acculturated to American traditions or norms.
   2) Intergenerational conflicts may occur around translation or interpretation.
   3) Family may use all other means of restoring health prior to seeking Western medical treatments.

continues

*Table 5* *continued*

## EXAMPLES OF CULTURAL INFLUENCES TO HEALTHCARE DECISIONS FOR CHILDREN

Mexicans

1) By behaving, working, and eating properly, illness may be prevented.

2) Good health may be related to good luck, and therefore good health is seen as a reward.

3) Illness may be seen as a punishment for wrongdoing by God, or it may be seen as caused by the supernatural.

Puerto Ricans

1) Evil spirits and other forces may be the cause of illness.

2) Causative theory of illness may be related to the theory of hot/cold.

3) May infrequently use modern healthcare systems; may seek counsel of spiritual medium.

*Lipson, Dibble, & Minarik. (1996).*
*http://eng.islam.ru/lib/pork*
*http://www.themodernreligion.com/misc/hh/pork.html*
*Hockenberry, M. (2005).*
*Wong, D. (2005).*

Resources to locate information on cultural diversity in pediatric healthcare:

Leininger, M., & McFarland, M. (2002). *Transcultural nursing: Concepts, theories, research and practice* (3rd ed.). New York: McGraw-Hill.

Linnard-Palmer, L., & Kools, S. (2004). Parents' refusal of medical treatment based on religious and/or cultural beliefs: The law, ethical principles, and clinical implications. *Journal of Pediatric Nursing, 19*(5), 351-355.

Linnard-Palmer, L., & Kools, S. (2005). Parents' refusal of medical treatment for cultural or religious beliefs: An ethnographic study on healthcare professionals' experiences. *Journal of Pediatric Oncology Nursing, 21*(6), 1-10.

Lipson, J., Dibble, S., & Minarik, P. (1996). *Culture and nursing care: A pocket guide.* San Francisco: UCSF Nursing Press.

Rosaldo, R. (1993). *Culture and truth: The remaking of social analysis* (2nd ed.). Boston: Beacon.

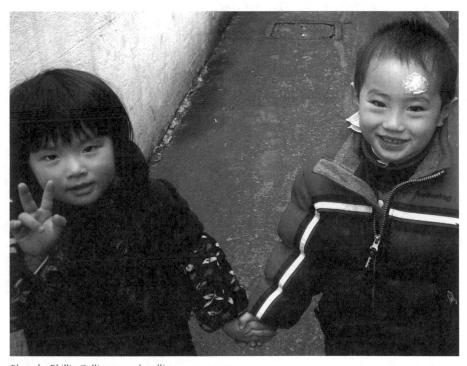

*Photo by Phillip Collier. www.thecollieragency.com.au*

6

# OVERVIEW OF PROFESSIONAL PERSPECTIVES

## PRINCIPLES OF PROFESSIONAL PRACTICE IN PEDIATRIC CARE

Healthcare professionals and those in related disciplines frequently hold membership in one or more professional organizations. Nursing and medicine have dozens of professional organizations that represent various specialties or interests. Some of these organizations take stances on politically charged social issues, while others limit their social policy work and specialize in educational and professional development. A review of the literature for position papers, suggestions, or opinions on the phenomena of medical treatment refusal or limitation for children, based on their parents' religious beliefs, found very few professional organizations that have made a statement or taken a stance on this topic. The American Academy of Pediatrics, American Medical Association, Christian Nurses Society, Association of Pediatric Oncology Nursing, Society of Pediatric Nurses, and Oncology Nursing Society have either published a viewpoint on the topic of treatment refusal based on religion or culture, or have published articles in their professional journals on the topic.

The following discussion discloses a variety of perspectives from members of three professional groups: nurses who have direct professional experiences with refusal phenomena, physicians, and journalists who follow nationwide stories on refusal scenarios, legal consequences for parents, and health outcomes for children. These discussions center on the professional perspectives of how much influence parents have on healthcare decisions for children.

# Perspectives of Healthcare Professionals

## Nurses

No nursing organization has published a position paper expressing views on this subject. A published article specially written to guide nurses in their roles, responsibilities, legal perspectives, or clinical standards on the topic of treat-

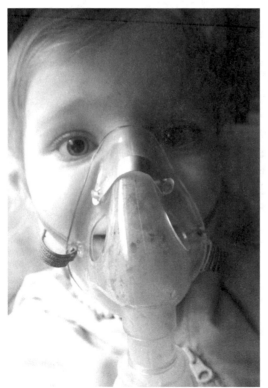

ment decisions could not be located after searching many electronic databases such as Medline, CINAHL, Proquest, Ebscohost, complementary medicine databases, and legal databases. Questioning nurse executives, nurse leaders, and directors of hospital operations on the subject of treatment refusal revealed no standardized policies, procedures, or clinical guidelines by these professionals.

At the time of this writing, this topic had been presented to 13 different professional organizations. At each of the sessions, whether a podium or a poster presentation,

*Photo by Dawn Allyn. www.dawnallyn.com*

dozens of nurses acknowledged the complexity of the topic and shared their personal experiences. Many of the nurses expressed concern not only for the well-being of the child, but also for the growing number of treatment refusal situations they have encountered as practicing nurses. The overarching theme in these informal discussions was that there simply is not enough information available to guide their practice and help them through these ethical dilemmas, or even to assist them with long-term feelings of moral distress.

## PHYSICIANS

It is not surprising that The American Academy of Pediatrics (AAP) takes a strong stand against religious exemptions to healthcare decisions for children—the AAP's mission is to attain optimal physical, mental, and social health and well-being for all infants, children, adolescents, and young adults. The AAP's Committee on Bioethics published guidelines in 1988 on religious exemptions from child abuse. The following is the opening quote:

> *The AAP's mission is to attain optimal physical, mental, and social health and well-being for all infants, children, adolescents, and young adults.*

> Children sometimes die or become disabled when they fail to receive medical treatment because of the strongly held religious or philosophical beliefs or practices of their parents. The numbers of such incidents of neglect are hard to ascertain reliably, but there are increasingly frequent reports in the mass media.

> We believe that the reported cases represent a much larger problem. (p. 169)

The AAP Committee on Bioethics offers guidelines, stating:

> The American Academy of Pediatrics recommends that all pediatricians, pediatric surgeons, and AAP state chapters vigorously take the lead to: (1) increase public awareness of the hazards to children growing out of religious exemptions to child abuse and neglect legislation; (2) support legislation in each state legislature to correct statutes and regulations that

permit harm to children under the shield of religious exemptions; (3) work with other child advocacy organizations and agencies to develop coordinated and concerted public and professional actions for revision of religious exemptions. The academy must unequivocally defend the rights of all children to the protection and benefits of the law and medicine when physical harm—or life itself—is in the balance. (American Academy of Pediatrics Committee on Bioethics, 1988, p. 170-171)

Another pertinent quote from the AAP (1988) states:

The Committee on Bioethics asserts: (1) the opportunity to grow and develop safe from physical harm with the protection of our society is a fundamental right of every child; (2) the basic moral principles of justice and of protection of children as vulnerable citizens require that all parents and caretakers must be treated equally by the laws and regulations that have been enacted by state and federal governments to protect children; (3) all child abuse, neglect, and medical neglect statutes should be applied without potential or actual exemption for religious beliefs; (4) no statute should exist that permits or implies that denial of medical care necessary to prevent death or serious impairment to children can be supported on religious grounds; (5) state legislatures and regulatory agencies with interests in children should be urged to remove religious exemptions clauses from statutes and regulations. (p. 170)

"Kids die from accidental deployment of air bags, and you get hearings in Congress. But this goes on [child deaths or injury from parents' refusal of medical care], and dozens die and people think there's no problem because the deaths happen one at a time. But the kids who die suffer horribly. This is Jonestown in slow motion" (Reaves, 2001, p. 1).

## PROFESSIONAL JOURNALISTS

Journalists have demonstrated an ongoing interest in locating and following the outcomes of pediatric medical treatment refusals. Although sometimes the articles may be interpreted as sensationalized, journalistic investigation has been shown to be fruitful in uncovering cases of neglect, abuse, and treatment refusal, as well as subsequent prosecution, acquittal, and other related legal consequences.

Joel Dyer, a writer for Colorado's *Boulder Weekly*, has researched the topic of parental refusal of medical care for religious preferences and has investigated both cults and well-established churches in America. In responding to the passage of Colorado House Bill 1286, which mandates criminal prosecution of people who withhold medical treatment from seriously ill children, Dyer (2000) wrote:

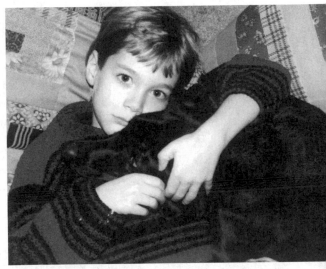

*Photo by Jane Palmer*

> I have to report that, as a rule, people like Amanda's parents [who prayed for their dying daughter instead of seeking medical care] actually love their children just as much as the rest of us love ours. They mourn the loss of children with equally sincere passion. People in faith-healing cults do what they do because they love their children, not because they are monsters. For a number of reasons, including what amounts to having been brainwashed by a cult, faith-healing adherents like Amanda's mom and dad are truly convinced that avoiding medical care is the best thing they can do for their kids. As much as we don't want to believe it's true, these people have no easier time watching their children die than the rest of us do. (para. 6)

Dyer (2000) wrote that the new law will likely not make much of a difference. He believes:

> The new law will not save a single child's life. Can we really expect people who have been brainwashed to the extent that they are willing to let the baby they love bleed to death in their arms from a simple wound to suddenly be motivated to seek medical care because they fear being charged with a crime? It's not likely. All this new law will accomplish is to put a small handful of grieving, misguided, brainwashed parents into prison and further radicalize and isolate the faith-healing cults that are actually responsible for the parent's contaminated thinking. And further isolating these cults will only make it more unlikely that deaths such as Amanda's will be prevented or even discovered. (para. 7)

*Oregon is among 43 states that still grant faith-healing congregational members immunities from child neglect and abuse prosecution*

Dyer (2000) further describes how many of these organizations exist on the fringes of society, promoting parents to home-school their children, thus making it even more difficult to locate and report these families to authorities. Dyer believes a bill like this will actually cause more children's deaths rather than stopping them, as those parents who have historically rushed their children to emergency rooms and hospitals for last-minute interventions will now fear prosecution.

Mark Larabee (1998), journalist for *The Oregonian*, wrote an article called "The Battle Over Faith Healing: When Prayer Pre-empts Medical Care." This article describes cases where children afflicted with medical conditions such as diabetes, Wilms' tumor, cystic fibrosis, or stomach cancer, or complications from prematurity, homebirths, and labor trauma, died while their parents upheld their religious convictions against seeking medical care and prayed for their children instead. He describes how Oregon is among 43 states that still grant faith-healing congregational members immunities from child neglect and abuse prosecution, and that Oregon is still one of only six states in the nation that grant immunity from murder, homicide, and manslaughter on the grounds of religious convictions. Larabee quotes one defending lawyer as saying: "Loving parents shouldn't be prosecuted for doing what they think is best for their children. It's not neglect if you actually believe it and you do what your religion says to do to get healed and you do it fervently. You can't prosecute religion away. It does not alter the religious practice. Outside of venting a public desire, it furthers no interest" (p. 4).

Journalist David Kostinchuk (2001) poses interesting questions. He asks, "Can faith healing be likened to torture?" He describes how the right to refuse medical treatment based on religious grounds is well-supported by many societies, when the individual is a consenting adult. But what happens when the individual is a child? He says the child denied medical treatment will most likely suffer "for very abstract reasons, which in all likelihood he or she does not understand" (p. 1). His expressed opinion is that this is not torture, but rather an extreme form of child abuse.

There is no single, overarching theme that has been developed by pediatric healthcare professionals to guide the practitioner through refusal scenarios. Nurses, physicians, and journalists vary on their views of pediatric treatment refusal, be it torture, child abuse, child neglect, religious brainwashing, group normative behaviors, misguided or misled behaviors, or simply faithful parents with distinct methods of conduct. It is quite justifiable for professional groups such as the Society of Pediatric Nurses or the American Academy of Pediatrics to develop and publish clinical practice guidelines.

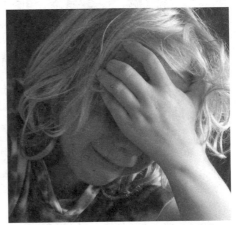

*Photo by Luc Sesselle. www.sxc.hu/profile/leonbidon*

# THEORETICAL INFLUENCES: DECISION-MAKING MODELS

The use of theory is beneficial in the interpretation of complex phenomena. Theory allows members of health science professions to view concepts and constructs as a way to make sense of, or make clear, elements of human response that are multifaceted. Ethical dilemmas have long been studied with the assistance of theoretical explanations.

Talking about the value of life when discussing the withholding of medical treatment can shed light on a parent's decision to refuse or withhold treatment. If parents' religious or cultural convictions are so strong they compel a conscious decision to apply the doctrine rather than sustain the life of their child, then viewing the value of the child's life becomes unclear. Vitalism—the doctrine that "vital forces" are active in living organisms, so that life cannot be explained solely by mechanism—as discussed by Paris (1982), is a theoretical construct that provides a perspective on the value of life: "Life is the ultimate value, and something that is to be preserved regardless of prognosis, regardless of cost, and regardless of social considerations" (p. 121). In contrast, parents with powerful religious convictions believe the application of religious law is by far more important than preserving life. An interview with a Jehovah's Witnesses nurse supports this conviction:

*Parents with powerful religious convictions believe that application of religious law is by far more important than preserving life.*

My relationship with God is paramount. My desire to ascend to His house is all encompassing to me. I would not, under any circumstance, ever, allow a blood transfusion to enter my veins, as this is God's law. It is clearly written in the Bible over and over ... you will not take blood into the body as blood is the very soul of life. I would not allow this law to be broken even in the situation where a physician tries to explain to me the need. No. Not ever. I love my God, and He loves me. I follow his word and his rules." (Personal communication, spring 2000)

According to Paris (1982): "We should always proceed with humility, with caution, with tentativeness, with a tilt to the side of life; with the understanding there is no such thing as life without value, that all life is valued as a gift of God and is precious in His eyes and hence, sacred for us; that whatever decision we make should be in the best interest of the child and not based on functional utility" (p. 144).

Kopelman, Irons, and Kopelman (1988) describe their findings from a descriptive survey conducted of 494 members (49% return rate) of the perinatal pediatric section of the AAP. The questionnaire contained general statements concerning the Baby Doe regulation, the federal regulation on the requirements to give all newborns maximal life-prolonging care. The majority of neonatologists who responded to the survey thought the current federal regulations were a mistake. After a detailed discussion, the authors posed several meaningful, unanswered questions, such as: Who should be included in the decision-making of the treatment dilemmas (i.e., the courts, solely the parents, physicians)? A standardized model for decision-making related to limiting or refusing medical treatments for children is not in the current literature.

*Do jury members or judges consider both the quality of life of the child, as well as the probability of recovery based on the feasibility of the treatments? Do decisions that make good sense to a judge make sound sense for the patient and the family? Who takes into account the religious doctrines that family members may hold so dear?*

Tierney, Weinberger, Greene, and Studdard (1984) surveyed 261 physicians who responded to a questionnaire concerning their reactions to the medico-legal and management problems of medical treatment refusal. Four case simulations were presented, and the respondents reported what they thought they would do in each situation. A wide variety of conflicting answers surfaced concerning the case of the child with sickle cell anemia in need of a blood transfusion: 72% of the respondents indicated they would have given the patient the blood transfusion after seeking a court order (100% of the pediatricians), 8% did not mention attempting to secure a court order, and 9% reported they would not have given the blood. Again, the conflict arises because of the lack of a normative decision-making process in this complex situation.

Paris (1982) analyzed the lack of a norm-less decision tree. "There are no guidelines, no principles for the physician's recommendations. They are simply ad hoc decisions and, as a result, they can be made quite poorly as easily as quite well" (p. 120). The author encouraged asking a series of important questions prior to definitive decision-making:

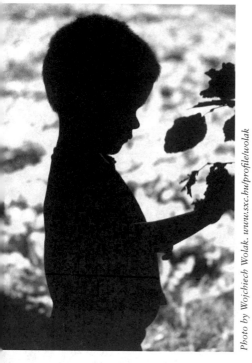

*Photo by Wojciech Wolak. www.sxc.hu/profile/wolak*

- What principles apply to such decisions?

- What type of ethical decision-making fits such cases?

- What are the facts?

- Do we have an actual factual basis?

After working to understand the answers to those questions: "We must examine the responses of the family and, because every response, every decision, is a value-laden one, we must try to discern what the values are. We must rank the operative values and then make the decision; looking to the past for guidance and, more important, to the future for the implications of the decision" (Paris, 1982, p. 120).

## DECISION-MAKING MODELS

Do jury members or judges consider both the quality of life of the child, as well as the probability of recovery based on the feasibility of the treatments? Do decisions that make good sense to a judge make sound sense for the patient and the family? Who takes into account the religious doctrines that family members may hold so dear? A review of the literature indicates long-term consequences of refusal episodes for children have not been investigated, and minimal references are available of the long-term consequences to the family as a unit. For example, Jon Watchko (1983) investigated the impact of decision making on infants who were critically ill and required treatment decisions. He published a theoretical discussion on a "two-schools of thought model": Should the responsibility of decision-making for critically ill infants fall to the hands of a forum (committee or courts), or should it fall to the hands of the parent and physician? Watchko proposed two questions: 1) Who should participate in this decision-making process? 2) With regard to individual participants, what degree of input should be expected and invited?

If these same questions raised by Watchko were posed about a religious family in crisis, regarding who will make the decisions about their child, research questions could be elaborated and restated as:

1) When faith crosses paths with children's health, who should participate in the treatment decisions?

2) With regard to individual participants such as clergy, church leaders, liaisons, family members, nurses, and physicians, how much information about one's faith should be invited as input?

Norman Fost, a pediatrician and medical ethicist, encourages placing the decision-making responsibility on a forum (committee or courts). He argues that an action can be considered right if it would be approved by one ideal observer with these five qualities (Fost, 1981):

1) omniscience (access to all relevant facts);

2) omnipercipience (ability to imagine the feelings of others vividly);

3) disinterest (having no vested interest in the situational outcomes);

4) dispassion (keeping emotions in check so as to not cloud critical thinking); and

5) consistency, as similar cases should be decided similarly (p. 795).

The problem is that the ideal situation rarely arises. More often, group consensus is reached with high hopes that as much information as possible was gathered and considered with each individual case of parental refusal of medical care. The committee would include membership from a multitude of professional disciplines—nursing, clergy, social services, medical, legal, and lay public. Fost further describes the concept of ideal observer as the one providing the platform for the decision-making process. It might be argued that when discussing the application of deeply rooted faith, the notion of being "observer" rather than involved party might be questionable. Fost describes how the greater the impartiality,

*When faith crosses paths with children's health, who should participate in the treatment decisions?*

the less chance "uncontested perception and self-interest of one party" will occur (Fost).

Another perspective in this first school of thought is the logical moral reasoning perspective provided by a multidisciplinary forum that values the preservation of life as being of paramount importance. The conflict experienced by parents or family desiring to follow the doctrine of their faith may surface when, like Jehovah's Witnesses believe, the treatment would possibly *damn the child's soul* (Watchko, 1983). This powerful outcome has the potential to alter the relationship between parent and child.

The second school of thought emphasizes parental input as the vital theme. S. Duff (Watchko, 1983) suggests the service given to families, with the aim of allowing them to evaluate largely on their own terms, would benefit from the input of the family members' views, contributions, and adaptations. He calls this process modified egalitarianism. Proponents of the second school of thought see this as placing the burdens of decision-making onto the family, because they are most familiar with the respective situation.

In previous literature, authors have proposed the notion that most parents actually use a committee, a "jury" if you will, to test the choices they plan to make or have made. This jury is made up of intimate friends, family members, clergy, neighbors, parishioners, and so on. This inherent jury already offers its views and support to the family. Families may or may not be consciously aware of their use of this inherent jury.

The final decision-making force may actually contain four assumptions:

1) The parents represent the noninstitutional perspective of the family and the child. As such, the parents' perspective is subjected to review by family members and pressure from various agencies, including the church and close friends.

2) The physician, even though he or she may be sympathetically engaged with the patient and family, primarily represents an institutional viewpoint. As such, the physician's viewpoint is subject to the constraints of peer review and pressure from other medical personnel, including nurses, social workers, and hospital administrators.

3) Hospital-based committees (interdisciplinary) would serve as consultants and advisors only, without authority to implement their decisions.

4) The courts, once involved in the decision-making process, would assume primary authority.

# EMOTIONAL REACTIONS AND MORAL DISTRESS IN REFUSAL SCENARIOS

The refusal of medical treatments for children is a highly complex phenomenon that can create profound emotional reactions for both staff and families. Emotional reactions can include fear, anguish, stress, anxiety, grief, tension, anger, and guilt. Although limited research has been conducted in the past on the impact of refusal episodes on those involved, the following reflects the impact of refusal scenarios on emotional well-being.

*Emotional reactions can include fear, anguish, stress, anxiety, grief, tension, anger, and guilt.*

## EMOTIONAL REACTIONS

The following list of families' and healthcare professionals' responses to refusal or limitation of medical treatment, with or without the loss of guardianship, demonstrates the variety of reasons of refusal and how emotionally charged they can be.

1) Families experience grief compounded by a report and investigation of possible medical neglect of their children (Kopelman et al., 1988).

2) Families of Jehovah's Witnesses may feel confusion, stress, loss of control, guilt, and, perhaps relief that the decision (transfusion therapy) is not or is no longer theirs to make (Anderson, 1983).

3) Forced treatment on competent patients comes via "forceful persuasion." Guilt may appear in relation to the patient's fears of having embarrassed the physician. Guilt may appear as expressed anger (Appelbaum & Roth, 1983).

4) The result of the violation of a deeply held, long-standing religious conviction can be devastating (Fox, 1990).

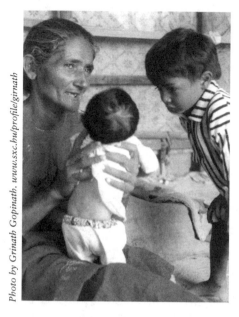

5) Those who hold religious beliefs that conflict with mainstream medical practice create a tension for clinicians who are attempting to honor the different religious perspectives of the individual and carry out what they believe to be their professional obligations (Lawry, Slomka, & Goldfarb, 1996).

6) The stress that nurses experience when involved with treatment decisions for Jehovah's Witnesses is discussed by Thurkauf (1989). Nurses are encouraged to verbalize their feelings, both to each other and as a group.

7) "Dilemmas are particularly complex when the patient involved is a child, not only because of the emotional nature of the situation, but also because of the uncertainty about who has moral and legal responsibility for authorization of treatment or withholding treatment" (Overbay, 1996, p. 19).

8) The concepts of "moral force" and "bilateral perceptions of being right" as discussed by Foreman (1999) support the professional/parent argument regarding decision-making about a child's medical treatment.

9) Advocates of forums, such as ethics committees and courts, describe reactions by parents such as denial, fear, anger, and guilt at the time when critical decisions may need to be made (Watchko, 1983).

## MORAL DISTRESS

Moral distress, as a concept, has had much attention in the health sciences literature. Moral distress has been defined as an emotional reaction one has toward emotionally painful or emotionally distressing situations. As medical technology evolves, as families represent unique cultural groups, as more and more ethical dilemmas arise, and as legal interventions continue to highly influence medicine, moral distress for healthcare professionals will continue to grow. Needless to say, individuals, families, and groups can all experience moral distress as involvement in complex, ethical dilemmas reaches beyond the patients themselves.

Moral distress has been described in several ways:

- "Moral distress is an experiential phenomenon of pained recognition that occurs in the human response pattern of valuing. It is multidimensional including combinations of physical, emotional, social and spiritual demands" (Hanna, 2001).

- Examples of moral distress include powerful reflections of unresolved emotions and unresolved emotional conflicts with families or physicians. Some nurses report moral distress is the outcome of unresolved conflicts (Pediatric Nursing Research Focus Group, personal communication, 2003).

- Three types of moral distress have been identified—shocked, muted, and chronic (dormant and unresolved; Hanna, 2001).

- Moral distress may occur when nurses are unable to translate their moral choices into moral action and when they are not included in the decision making (Perkin, Young, Freier, Allen, and Orr, 1997).

- In moral distress, a nurse knows the morally right course of action to take, but institutional structures and conflicts with co-workers create obstacles (Jameton, 1993).

The following describes moral distress as it relates to participation in ethical dilemmas:

- The professional role one plays leads to differences in moral action, not in ethical reasoning or moral motivation (Corley, Elswick, & Gorman, 2001).

- The Moral Distress Scale (Corley et al.) has 32 items on a 7-point Likert scale. A factor analysis yielded three variations of moral distress: individual responsibility, not in the patient's best interest, and deception.

- Moral distress was found to be associated with anger and frustration, leading to burnout of experienced nurses (Sundin-Huard & Fahy, 1999).
- Moral distress was found to be associated with the inability to translate moral choices into moral action (Perkin et al., 1997).

Coping with moral distress is typically unique to the individual. One individual may carry moral distress for a long time. The distress may compound with each new situation, leading to departure from professional practice. Others may be far more able to adjust with each "dose" of moral distress and carry on with strength.

*There is a lot of moral conflict, especially in peds where they [the children] don't have a voice, but when you silence the parents then, as a nurse, you feel you have to be the voice; but your voice is muffled because you are on the medical-team side.*

*— Pediatric nurse*

7

# ETHNOGRAPHIC RESEARCH IN TREATMENT REFUSAL CASES

## ETHNOGRAPHY AS A MEANS OF STUDYING HUMAN BEHAVIOR

Ethnography is a good way to explore human behavior and cultural exchanges. The application of religious beliefs in the healthcare setting is seen as a form of cultural exchange. Further, each healthcare setting is made up of unique factors that contribute to a unique cultural context. Ethnography is a way to discover and explore the cultural exchanges that take place among healthcare professionals, families, clergy, and children.

## WHAT IS MEANT BY THE METHODOLOGY OF ETHNOGRAPHY?

Ethnography and ethnonursing (Leininger & McFarland, 2002) are one way to study culture. Culture is a learned, adaptive, and shared way within groups of people with identifiable patterns, symbols, and material and nonmaterial data. Culture has biological, physical, spiritual, and historical features nurses should know and understand. Culturally congruent and beneficial nursing care can only occur when healthcare values, expressions, or patterns are known and used explicitly for appropriate, safe, and meaningful care. According to Leininger and Mcfarland, knowledge of how to provide medically safe and culturally congruent, responsible, and sensitive care is lacking. Cultural conflicts, imposition practices, stresses, and pain are the consequences of this knowledge deficit.

Ethnography is inductive, scientific, investigative, and rigorous, and emphasizes the perspectives of people in the research setting. Ethnography takes the position that behavior and the ways in which people construct and make meaning of their worlds and their lives are highly variable and locally specific (those that originate in and are found in one specific location). Ethnography assumes that one must first discover what people actually do and the reasons they give for doing it. The researcher enters as an invited guest, using self as the data collection instrument, and uses keen eyesight and hearing to discover, learn the meaning of, and steer away from any control that would influence the integrity of the local culture. The product is an interpretive story, reconstruction, or narrative about a group of people that includes their history; therefore, it paints a picture of people going about their daily lives, in the course of living out those daily lives, over a period of time. The final goal of applied ethnographic research is to understand sociocultural problems and use these understandings to bring about positive change in communities, institutions, or groups (LeCompte & Schensul, 1999).

*Culture mediates between human beings and chaos: It influences what people perceive and guides people's interactions with each other.*

One of the many definitions of culture is that it is a system of symbols that are shared, learned, and passed on through generations of a social group. Culture mediates between human beings and chaos: It influences what people perceive and guides people's interactions with each other. Culture is a process rather than a static entity, and it changes over time (Lipson, Dibble, and Marinik, 1996).

Although there is considerable variety regarding prescription and practice, ethnography involves the ethnographer participating, overtly and covertly, in people's daily lives for an extended period of time while watching, listening, asking questions, and collecting data. The object is to throw light on the issues that are the focus of the research, all the time identifying the routine ways in which people make sense of their world in everyday life. The value of ethnography, as a social research method, is founded upon the existence of variations in cultural patterns across and within societies and their significance for understanding social processes. Even when the researcher is studying a familiar group or setting, the participant observer is required to treat the group as "anthropologically strange," in an effort to make explicit the presuppositions he or she takes for granted as a member of the culture. In this way, it is hoped the culture is turned into an object available for study. Naturalism rests on the proposition that it is possible to construct an account of the culture under investigation that both understands it from within and captures it as external to, and independent of, the researcher—in other words, it is an approach that recognizes culture as a natural phenomenon with social rules and cultural beliefs (Hammersley & Atkinson, 1995).

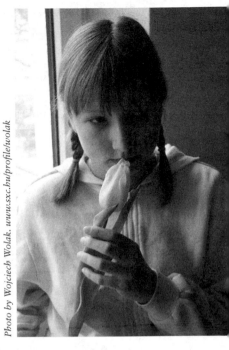

*Photo by Wojciech Wolak. www.sxc.hu/profile/wolak*

Ethnography involves an ongoing attempt to place specific encounters, events, and understandings into a fuller, more meaningful context. Research design, fieldwork, and various methods of inquiry combine to produce historically, politically, and personally situated accounts, descriptions, interpretations, and representations of human lives.

Ethnography is both a process and a product. The experience is meaningful, and human behavior is generated from, and informed by, this meaningfulness. The pioneers of ethnography experienced fieldwork as not merely a rite of passage, but rather as a lived reality that was the center of their intellectual and emotional lives (Denzin & Lincoln, 2000).

## WHAT IS MEANT BY THE METHODOLOGY OF ETHNOGRAPHIC INQUIRY?

As was mentioned earlier, ethnography is an inductive, scientific, investigative, and rigorous process that focuses on the perspectives of the people in the research setting. The ethnographer takes the position that behavior and the ways in which people construct and make meaning of their worlds and their lives are highly variable and locally specific (those that originate in and are found in one specific location). The ethnographer assumes s/he must first discover what people actually do and the reasons they identify for doing things.

The goal of applied ethnographic research is to provide an understanding of sociocultural problems and use these understandings to bring about positive change in communities, institutions, or groups (LeCompte & Schensul, 1999).

1) Ethnography and ethnonursing seek to study culture. Culture, being a learned, adaptive, and shared way of people with identifiable patterns, symbols, and material and nonmaterial data, has biological, physical, spiritual, and historical features that nurses can know and understand.

2) Culturally congruent and beneficial nursing care can only occur when healthcare values, expressions, or patterns are known and used explicitly for appropriate, safe, and meaningful care. Cultural conflicts, cultural imposition practices, cultural stresses, and cultural pain reflect the lack of culture-care knowledge needed by healthcare professionals to provide culturally congruent, responsible, safe, and sensitive care (Leininger & McFarland, 2002).

3) Culture may be defined as a system of symbols that are shared, learned, and passed on through generations of a social group. Culture links human beings and chaos—it is the basis of what people perceive and what guides people's interactions with each other. It is a process rather than a static entity, and it changes over time (Lipson et al., 1996).

4) Ethnography involves the ethnographer participating, overtly and covertly, in people's daily lives for an extended period of time, watching, listening, asking questions, and collecting data. The object is to

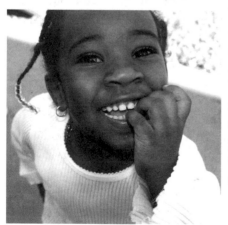

throw light on the issues that are the focus of the research, all the time identifying the routine ways in which people make sense of the world in everyday life. The value of ethnography as a social research method is founded upon the existence of such variations in cultural patterns across and within societies, and their significance for understanding social process (Hammersley & Atkinson, 1995).

*Photo by Anissa Thompson. www.anissat.com/photos.php*

5) Ethnography involves an ongoing attempt to place specific encounters, events, and understandings into a fuller, more meaningful context. As a result, research design, fieldwork, and various methods of inquiry to produce historically, politically, and personally situated accounts, descriptions, interpretations, and representations of human lives are combined. Ethnography is both a process and a product. The experience is meaningful, and human behavior is generated from and informed by this meaningfulness. The pioneers of ethnography experienced fieldwork not merely as a rite of passage, but rather the lived reality that was the center of their intellectual and emotional lives (Denzin & Lincoln, 2000.)

Ethnographic methodology is an excellent fit for the investigation of cultural exchanges between healthcare providers and families whose religious and cultural beliefs influence healthcare decisions for children. The following sections present a discussion of how the application of ethnographic methods was used to explore these cultural exchanges.

# TREATMENT REFUSAL PERSPECTIVES OF HEALTHCARE PROFESSIONALS*

## INTRODUCTION

Pediatric nurses working in urban settings where ethnic and cultural diversity are commonplace may encounter families whose belief systems are at odds with Western medical treatment decisions for their acutely ill children. Both cultural and religious beliefs can impact whether or not parents seek medical attention, consent to modern medical treatment, or attempt to refuse or limit healthcare. A review of the literature revealed descriptions of many reasons for treatment refusal, but minimal research on the impact of treatment refusal on bedside interactions between the nurse and the family during subsequent

*Pages 111-128 adapted from Linnard-Palmer, L., & Kools, S. (2005), Parents' refusal of medical treatment for cultural or religious beliefs: An ethnographic study of healthcare professionals' experiences. *Journal of Pediatric Oncology Nursing*, 22(1), 48-57. Copyright SAGE Publications, Thousand Oaks, CA. All rights reserved. Used with permission

care interventions. As immigration rates continue to grow and urban populations explode, and as church memberships continue to increase at high rates, pediatric nurses will encounter a wide array of cultural and religious beliefs on a more frequent basis. The purpose of this section is to present the findings of an ethnographic study that supported the investigation of healthcare professionals' experiences with parental refusal of medical treatment for acutely ill children.

When families refuse medical treatment for cultural or religious reasons, a variety of processes and conclusions may occur. Healthcare teams may attempt to negotiate with the family concerning treatment for acutely ill children. When negotiation or educational attempts prove unsuccessful in obtaining parental consent, healthcare professionals may request an ethics committee consultation. If the child's condition is unstable and expeditious treatments are required, the healthcare team may seek temporary legal guardianship (mandated by state law) to administer the recommended medical interventions. Not all parental treatment limitation or refusal decisions require these ethics committee or state guardianship procedures. Sometimes the parents want to have their beliefs heard and acknowledged, or they want to delay treatment so prayer sessions or cultural practices can be performed. Ethnographic research has demonstrated that each refusal episode is unique and requires individualized considerations and actions.

## Pediatric Oncology

Pediatric oncology nurses work in an area that requires numerous interventions that may be seen as incongruent with various religious and cultural beliefs and frameworks. Children who are diagnosed with oncology or hematology problems frequently need blood transfusions or blood products. As was addressed earlier, Jehovah's Witnesses allow only very specific blood products (see Table 3, page 73). When children of Jehovah's Witnesses are diagnosed with oncology or hematology problems, the family may be faced with critical treatment decisions. Christian Scientists, who prefer prayer as a first or sole intervention before traditional medical interventions are applied, may find themselves in conflict with lengthy chemotherapy courses of treatment. Fundamentalist Christians, or families whose church doctrines encourage lengthy prayer sessions, may find themselves in conflict when tumor growth is exponential and treatment is urgent. Vegan (those who refuse to use or consume any animal products) Black Muslims may be confronted with the need to

112

increase oral protein intake or may be faced with the administration of beef- or pork-based pharmaceutical agents.

## RELIGIOUS FRAMEWORKS

More than 31 churches have been dentified in the literature as having doc- trines, religious frameworks, or teachings that include limitation, refusal, or preference for prayer over traditional Western medical interventions. When families, clergy, and healthcare professionals encounter diversity in beliefs, the sharing, negotiating, and personal exchanges that occur result in one of several probable outcomes. These outcomes may leave children in the middle to inter- pret the struggle in their own way and according to their developmental level.

## CULTURAL FRAMEWORKS

Cultural affiliations have been known to influence treatment decisions for par- ents of acutely ill children. Nurses and other groups have identified members of Islamic Muslim, Black Muslim, Hindu, Jewish, and Native American Indian cultural groups as having beliefs that may influence treatment decisions.

## EMOTIONAL IMPACT

The literature contains descriptions of a variety of emotional responses to the refusal of medical treatment for children. Both family members and healthcare workers may experience tension during decision making. Parents may expe- rience grief that is compounded by their fears or reactions to possible child abuse or medical neglect charges (Kopelman, Irons, and Kopelman, 1988). Parents may elect to leave the hospital or emergency department against medical ad- vice (AMA) in response to either the prob- ability of a child abuse report or attempts to persuade them to consent for treatment. Parents may feel confusion, stress over loss of control, guilt, and even some relief dur- ing state-mandated treatment when medical decisions are not, or are no longer, theirs to make (Anderson, 1983). Lawry, Slomka, and Goldfarb (1996) describe how these conflicts with mainstream medical practitio- ners can create tension for clinicians when

*Conflicts with main- stream medical practi- tioners can create tension for clinicians when they try to honor different re- ligious perspectives while carrying out what they believe to be obligations of their profession.*

they try to honor different religious perspectives while carrying out what they believe to be the obligations of their profession.

Nurses who have been taught to honor family perspectives and wishes, and who have been taught that family advocacy is paramount, may feel conflicted when they are asked to participate in mandated treatment to enforce medical prescriptions against parents' wishes. The literature contains descriptions of the moral distress experienced by neonatal nurses who work with families that have strong desires concerning treatment decisions. Other reactions, as described by Thurkauf (1989), include stress related to treatment decisions. In situations where the patient is a child, the emotional nature of treatment refusals during the complex dilemma is particularly difficult when linked with the uncertainty about who is responsible for the moral and legal implications of the child's experiences and outcomes (Overbay, 1996). This chapter presents two treatment-refusal ethnographic studies. The central idea of Study #1 was to investigate pediatric healthcare professionals' reported emotional and biophysical reactions to the impact of these powerfully complex human interactions. Study #2 focuses on the perspectives of families, church communities, and clergy.

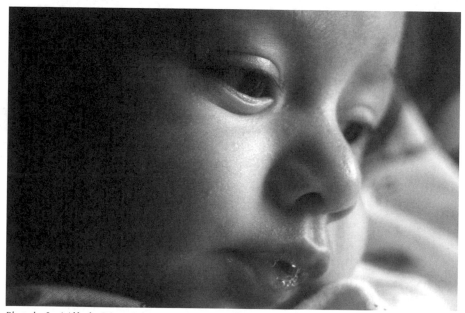

*Photo by José Alfredo Gómez Soberano. www.sxc.hu/profile/krake*

Because little is known about experiences associated with parental refusal or limitation of medical treatments for children hospitalized for acute or chronic illnesses, ethnographic methodology was used to investigate the phenomenon.

# STUDY #1

## RESEARCH QUESTIONS:

1) What is the impact of parental religious beliefs on the interactions between family members and the healthcare team during decision-making regarding the medical treatment of the acutely ill child?

2) What are the processes and outcomes of medical treatment refusal, including loss of guardianship, from the perspectives of nurses?

3) What is the impact of mandated treatment against parents' beliefs and wishes on health state, stress level, and functional status of the nurses involved?

## RESEARCH METHODS

An ethnographic design was used to investigate the experiences of pediatric nurses working in one large acute care facility. Pediatric nurses were defined as a cultural group based on their unique set of practices, behaviors, and methods of communication. Both in-depth interviews and field notes were acquired to capture the cultural phenomenon of parental refusal as described in the experiences and perspectives of the nurses. Twenty nurses were interviewed individually, and field notes of witnessed accounts of refusal scenarios were recorded over the course of 18 weeks.

## SAMPLE

The sample population of the study was obtained through the use of convenience nonprobability sampling procedures. After obtaining written permission from a representative of the nursing administration at a large urban, acute care hospital facility and approval by the University of California, San Francisco's Institutional Review Boards Committee on Human

Research, a flier was posted in the pediatric nurses' lounge and in the report room. The primary investigator also verbally solicited volunteer participants over a period of 2 weeks by explaining the purpose of the study to nurses on each shift. Following a description of the purpose and procedures of the study, as well as articulation of potential risks, all participants were asked to sign a letter of consent. Networking and snowballing procedures (asking individuals for further referrals) were also used to obtain a representative sample of 20 pediatric nurses.

The sample represented several interesting demographic variables. All of the participants were female. The mean age of the nurses was 32 and spanned from the early 20s to the early 50s. The length of pediatric nursing practice ranged from 2 years to more than 27 years, and educational preparation ranged from associate degree to current enrollment in doctoral education. The nurses represented several ethnic and racial backgrounds, including Filipino (10%), Hispanic (10%), Iranian (5%), African-American (5%), and Caucasian (70%). This varied sample was not solicited, but rather reflects the diversity found in the Greater San Francisco Bay Area.

## THE SETTING

The setting of the study was a large pediatric unit situated in a predominantly adult acute-care facility located in the San Francisco Bay Area. Pediatric oncology and hematology patients, ranging from early infancy to late adolescence, comprised 60% of the average daily census of the unit. Other diagnoses included children hospitalized for surgical procedures, congenital disorders, infectious diseases, and acute episodes of chronic disorders. The patient population came from urban areas and included a variety of economic levels.

## THE RESEARCH INSTRUMENT

The researcher (a veteran acute-care pediatric nurse) administered a set of open-ended, probing questions that elicited narratives. Although all interviews were based on an interview guide, the researcher adapted the voicing and sequence of the questions with each subsequent interview to maximize disclosure and explore each participant's recorded interviews for data saturation. No second interviews were conducted, as each transcribed interview was deemed complete.

## THE INTERVIEWS

After obtaining verbal consent on the phone, participants were interviewed in quiet, confidential locations of their choice. Locations for interviews included coffee shops, classrooms on an academic campus, parks, and offices. Formal written consent was obtained just prior to data collection after a full description of the aim of the study. The interviews ranged from 45 minutes to more than 2 hours.

For each interview, a trusting rapport was quickly developed, supported by professional experiences shared by the interviewer and the participants. On several occasions, the researcher steered participants away from asking questions about the researcher's personal patient and family experiences and views. Several of the participants expressed an interest in the researcher's opinions of refusal scenarios that were described. As the researcher became more experienced with interview techniques, deeper and more disclosive narrations were elicited that subsequently produced more profound and intense personal reflection.

Field notes were taken during the data collection period. The purpose of the field notes was to describe the refusal episodes witnessed, the mood and environment for each interview, and the impact of the research process on the researcher. Field notes were analyzed at a later date as a means of further confirmation and elaboration of themes identified in the findings.

Sixteen of the 20 interviews were audiotaped for future transcribing. Four participants refused to be audiotaped. The tapes were carefully reviewed for clarity and for remembrance of the emotional state of the participant during key times of disclosure.

Interviews were open coded without regard for relative importance in an effort to expand the data to determine the breadth of possible themes. Data were then limited through the development of salient categories that grouped related concepts into broad themes.

Data from both the interviews and field notes were analyzed using traditional ethnographic methods, which included:

1) explication of culture through gradual thickening of symbolic webs of meaning (Rosaldo, 1993);

2) covert and overt participation in people's lives over time, watching what happens, listening to what is said, and asking questions (Hammersley & Atkinson, 1995); and

3) repositioning, or changes of perceptions, of researchers as they go about understanding other cultures (Rosaldo, 1993).

## FIELD EXPERIENCES

Ethnographic field notes are written responses of the investigator regarding the experience of data collection. The notes include descriptions of environments, communication patterns, emotional responses, and other signi-ficant spoken and unspoken information pertinent to the development of the research findings. Ethnography, the study of cultural patterns, is captured by a variety of data collection means; field notes substantiate the data.

The investigator was also able to witness three refusal scenarios during the data collection period. Extensive field notes were created after the events.

Field notes allowed for documentation of the communication patterns that occurred and provided a source of confirmation of the themes identified during subsequent interviews.

## FINDINGS AND DISCUSSION

Interpretive narrative analysis of transcriptions and field notes uncovered a variety of social and cultural circumstances of the treatment refusal. Participants revealed three types of refusal scenarios:

1) A child is brought in by parents with a medical condition directly linked to or attributed to the parents' cultural or religious-based health practices.

   Examples disclosed in the data: Untreated communicable diseases for which immunizations are available, infections, sepsis, and diet-related cases of severe anemia.

   This is the greatest of the power struggles ... vivid ... physicians use threats and the parents stay unreasonable. ... This is the most emotionally charged situation.

> When I have encountered a family whose kid was sick because of their choices, not ours, I felt sick ... you know, like I want to fight with them and tell them how I feel, yet I also want to educate them on what it is all about ... you know, how to not let this happen again. ... I just have to ask myself, is religion worth a little kid suffering?

> I had this one little guy with failure to thrive, anemia because of some beliefs around food. Now ... who can let that happen? ... just a little guy.

2) A child develops a treatable medical condition that was not the consequence of the family's cultural health practices or religious beliefs, yet the family's religious or cultural belief system did not allow them to agree to a curative treatment.

Examples disclosed in the data include chemotherapy for early stages of retinoblastoma and blood products for severe anemia associated with vaso-occlusive episodes related to sickle cell disease.

> It was retinoblastoma, but anyway, they didn't want treatment for her even though it was curable and we were trying to tell them this is, like, a very easy way to cure this thing. ... At the most she might lose her eye, but maybe not, you know, it is not going to spread yet anyway ... and they were very adamant that it was against their beliefs to treat it.

One nurse described the aftermath of parents losing authority to make treatment decisions for their child:

> Sometimes there is a struggle and ambivalence that parents have in trying to comply with religious beliefs in the face of great potential sacrifice (i.e., losing legal guardianship or losing their child to a medical condition). ... Maybe sometimes it is a win-win because the parents' consciences might be clear. ... They did not voluntarily violate their church laws. ... Their child can be cured or treated by the prohibited treatment.

3) A child is brought to a physician suffering from a severe medical condition that has a dismal prognosis. The parents continue to refuse medical treatment and, at times, symptom management, even at the risk of losing guardianship to the state based on medical neglect.

Examples disclosed in the data include progressive, high-risk, acute lymphocytic leukemia; metastasizing osteogenic or Ewing's sarcomas; and rapidly growing lymphomas.

> I don't know. ... When the child's disease is probably going to take them, then I can understand why parents do this, but ... if there is a chance of survival or cure, then the state has to come in and intervene. One mom refused any treatment for her 10-year-old's leukemia because he had had a brain tumor when he was younger. ... They think all the treatment he received back then caused him to develop the leukemia now. ... Because the child's state might respond to chemo, the doctors got guardianship of him and he got treated for weeks.

Within the context of these types of refusal scenarios, the three central themes of the nurses' experiences were identified as:

1) weathering the storm of moral conflict;

2) closeness and involvement versus distance and retreat; and

3) unresolved battles between supportive and oppositional villages.

These three main themes were developed from an in-depth analysis of the data that started immediately after the first interview and continued during all subsequent data collection. The major theme of weathering the storm, identified in all 20 interviews, was disclosed in the descriptions of how powerful the refusal situation was on influencing communication patterns. The influence was found in communications between the nurses and the families, leading to stressful interactions, experiences of moral distress and conflict, and ongoing attempts to negotiate treatment decisions.

*Nurses described how they did not have the opportunity or the means to learn about the religious doctrines during or after the storm.*

## Weathering the Storm of Moral Conflict

Nurse participants uniquely described entering into, existing within, and leaving a storm of conflict and emotional upheaval during the refusal scenario and its eventual resolution. Nurses described how calm most interactions were within typical family and child acute-care situations. In contrast, a storm occurred during medical treatment refusal events, especially when the parents' religious beliefs conflicted with the nurses' spiritual or philosophical framework, or the child was at risk for severe harm from withholding treatment. The storm is created by intense dissonance between the views of the parents and the nurses. During this difficult period, nurses must navigate effective care for the child and also self-care, seeing the ethical dilemma as a real source of moral distress.

> Well, us older nurses have seen this many times. Sometimes it is just like walking into a black cloud ... you know, like a storm, and them trying to navigate the whole thing through. I don't think you can get any larger of an ethical dilemma. ... Who knows what really to do and how to think?

> I think that time heals the tension. ... But, meanwhile I just concentrate on the needs of the child, even if the parents are upset, turn their backs on me, stomp out of the room. ... I just keep my focus on the child.

Often the nurses stated the storm never became calm. Instead, they felt a lack of resolution and expressed confusion surrounding the legal factors.

> I listen. ... I grit my teeth. ... I stay involved, but I really wish I knew more about my rights ... my legal responsibilities ... whose side am I supposed to be on?

Sometimes the nurses do not know how much of their
emotions are expressed during their silence with the parents. ... They use silence because they are afraid to say
anything that might get them in trouble, you know, with
the law and all. ... They just go in and do the treatment
and get out, unsure of what their legal roles are.

Nurses described how they did not have the opportunity or the means
to learn about the religious doctrines during or after the storm. The desire
to learn more about various religious frameworks and cultural beliefs that
influence parental decision-making was expressed by all the nurse participants. Learning more specific religious and cultural information was identified as a potential way to resolve nurses' emotional upheaval.

I think that what is missing is that in nursing training,
not just curriculum, but when you go to the hospital, you
are not prepared for it. I have always wondered why we
didn't have a better training in terms of culture, religion
and legal stuff ... what to say and, like, what to expect,
and where I can look stuff up. ... How can I approach this
without a knowledge base?

## CLOSENESS AND INVOLVEMENT VERSUS DISTANCE AND RETREAT

Several nurses talked about how they made conscious and unconscious
decisions concerning their level of involvement with the families and the
refusal situation. They described a continuum of involvement that ranged
from jumping in right away and staying with the assignment (some described primary nurse assignments) to refusing to care for the child and
family at all (some described needing to negotiate this with their professional peers). Some nurses felt the need to retreat from their patient care
responsibilities as soon as possible, either by requesting a change in their
patient assignment or by coming in before their shift to ensure that their
assignment would not include the family.

Oh yeah, the religious thing, boy that is something
I try to avoid. I just tend to avoid it all. ... They get so

> over-controlling about their kid while following their
> faith. ... That is the biggest conflict I can think of in my
> work. It is so hard for me to try to offer them my help;
> the whole blame thing starts. ... I just tend to avoid the
> conflict. ... I get these preconceived ideas of these families,
> and I automatically say, "I am out of here."

> Sometimes I just step back, just to get out for a while,
> when it ... when it gets to be all just too much to handle.

A few of the nurses described the opposite of retreat and explained how they became devoted to influencing the conflict situation by being present, advocating for the child's needs, and involving outside support such as social services, child life or play therapists, pastoral care, or nursing supervisors and administrators.

> I think that you at some point ... it is very hard to distance
> yourself, either when you agree with the family's perspec-
> tives or at least you start really seeing it their way ... or you
> start feeling like you see it from the medical way. ... When
> there is no alternative, I might try to advocate a lot more
> and spend much more time with that family explaining the
> signs and symptoms of what is happening with their child.
> ... But when I think that the medical team is just trying to
> get another statistic, to put someone into a study, then I do
> feel like I am siding with the family. ... It is really tough.

Requesting assistance from the institution's ethics committee was discussed by only two nurses. When others were probed on this topic, some said it never occurred to them that the ethics committee would be on their side or see the situation from the nurses' perspectives.

Participants shared their understanding of the parents' positions as well:

> And I think that it is a really hard position for parents to
> be in because they feel isolated from their child. They feel
> like they are no longer the controllers of their own kids. It
> is a loss, at some level, of being the child's parent.

## Unresolved Battles Between the Supportive and Oppositional Villages

Several of the nurses described the continuing conflict they have as they have thought about the unresolved clashes and divergent emotions generated between members of the healthcare team and the family. One theme identified was that of opposing groups whose goals and foci were in opposition, with the healthcare team being identified as the oppositional village and the family unit and support systems being the supportive village.

The healthcare team focused on the need for treatment and traditional care for the child at all costs, and the family, clergy, and neighbors focused on the integrity of the belief systems of the parents. One assumption made by the researcher was that these villages would have definite borders or boundaries. This assumption was consistently invalidated by the participants. Some nurses identified with the supportive village, and some family constellations had internal conflicts, such as one parent in agreement with the religious or cultural belief, and the other parent in disagreement.

> There is always such confusion and anger from both sides. We impose on them, and it confuses the families who don't really understand the numbers very well [referring to offered statistical probabilities of the child's projected outcome]. ... I think our system is really biased towards what the medical team thinks and what they want, and they make it clear to the families that they will win in court.

> My biggest challenge has been to find a middle ground, trying not to seem biased and still seeming like I care about the family, and yet still maintain my employment by not going too far against the medical team and their persistence. ... So you just have to walk that fine line.

> You just have to keep on trying to persuade them (the families) that you are doing the right thing ... until the kid's treatment is done, they leave, or they die. ... You just have to keep trying to persuade them, even if they are exploding in your face.

It is very clear to me now that you are not supposed to say anything against the medical team. ... The message is very clear. You are supposed to advocate for your patients, but not in a way that would in any way put down what the medical team is putting forth.

The nurses can just feel as though they are useless, that they have no role, not really on either side, just caught in the middle.

Not all of the research participants shared the experience of parents temporarily losing guardianship to the state for mandated treatments. Those who were involved in the process of temporary guardianship, or at least witnessed the process of securing temporary guardianship, shared the varied responses of the families:

So they [physicians] went to court, and it seemed that when the court order came, they [parents] almost felt everything was out of their hands; they tried their best to uphold their religion and now they couldn't do anything. ... They were not mad initially ... but once the treatment started ... Oh my God, I had to get out of there fast.

I have seen both extremes. ... Either the family was relieved when the court order for blood was received and there was nothing more they could do ... or they were yelling mad when one kid was forced to get chemo when the situation was based on no record of a child ever being cured ... no statistical evidence and still being forced to get chemotherapy and the families being dragged through the process and then not coming back for second and third rounds of chemo ... which is worse than never having gotten chemo to begin with because you start the process and you don't end it ... you don't finish it. ... One family just took off and left for Mexico.

In a way you listen to these doctors do it and it just sounds like coercion. ... They told them: "We can go get a court order, and it will just take longer, and in the mean-

time your child's hemoglobin will just continue to drop. ...
She could get sicker. ... It is up to you whether you want
to give it [blood] sooner or have her deteriorate and give
it later."

## MORAL DISTRESS

Moral distress was described by several of the nurses as an outcome of the
communication process during the refusal event. The term moral distress
was used by several of the nurses, and others described the event as "emotional distress" and "ethical despair."

> Moral distress ... that is it. I would define it as a conflict
> between what you know is right and wrong and what is
> happening and ... um ... there is definitely a lot of that in
> these situations.

> I felt it. There were families who refused treatment, and
> I felt that it was their right to refuse it, and I felt that it
> was not in the best interest of the child to receive it [treat-
> ment], so I felt moral distress ... in the sense that I agreed
> with the family, and I felt moral distress with my medi-
> cal team. ... They push the drugs, but it's me who carries
> out the plan. ... They just write it and go home. ... But
> me, the one who puts it inside their child, [is] gowned up
> with gloves, and the parents [asking] me, "Why are you
> so gowned up? ... You are putting poison into my child!"
> ... I have to poison the kid's whole body and then rescue
> parts of it and give the supportive care. ... You just feel
> like the bad hand. ... That is what is distressing.

> I feel there is a lot of moral conflict, especially in peds
> where they [the children] don't have a voice, but when
> you silence the parents then, as a nurse, you feel you have
> to be the voice; but your voice is muffled because you
> are on the medical-team side. ... It is very hard. I think as
> a nurse you protect yourself from the moral distress by
> choosing your patients, calling in early, giving the emo-
> tionally hard patients to the new grads.

## LONG-TERM CONSEQUENCES

The nurses infrequently disclosed lasting or long-term effects of the refusal events on their health, stress level, or functional status. Because of the nurses' lengthy and direct involvement during the treatment-refusal episodes, and because of the complexity of most situations disclosed, the researcher assumed there would be long-term consequences on the well-being of the nurse. That, however, proved not to be the case as nurses did not identify treatment refusal scenarios as having a lasting, negative impact on their lives. Nurses did indicate long-term concern for the health of the family unit after refusal situations.

> I wonder about the future. ... What is the result of this episode? ... Do the parents ever question their own beliefs? ... Or are their children not eligible for the spiritual rewards promised to the faithful? ... Could there be lasting resentment towards the Big Brother who stepped in and usurped their parental authority and autonomy? ... What happens during the next episode?

## SUMMARY OF FINDINGS

Parent refusal of medical treatment will continue to emerge in the discipline of pediatric practice as church membership grows and as medical technology continues to expand. As healthcare professionals are expected to provide state-of-the-art medical technology with a philosophical belief that saving lives is paramount above all else, families will be expected to agree and consent to use these technologies to treat their children's illnesses. This difference of beliefs has led to battles, some with resolution and others not. Until nurses understand the incongruity between religious and cultural convictions and available technology, the battle will continue, and bedside interactions will continue to be strained.

The effect of this moral and ethical dilemma on role processes and communication patterns was clearly demonstrated in the interviews with the nurses. Some nurses simply stayed away from the situations of refusal. Others, whose involvement level varied, attempted to secure their role as patient and parent advocate while balancing their legal role of preventing medical neglect or not promoting medical neglect. Nurses either battled with the families whose religious or cultural frameworks differed from their own, attempted to balance the diverse views, or kept silent.

A complete analysis determined there are no clear guidelines published or available to nurses, or to other pediatric healthcare professionals, on appropriate bedside conduct during conflicts. Nor are there clear guidelines as to how nurses should maintain a supportive relationship with families during medical-refusal scenarios.

## Clinical Application of Research Findings

Nurses can have a stronger leadership role if they apply cultural knowledge to strained communications at the bedside. Learning more about the impact of culture and religion on healthcare decisions can increase cultural sensitivity and maintain functioning relationships with family units.

Healthcare professionals need to be aware of how ethical dilemmas impact their day-to-day functioning as acute care nurses. The goal of this explorative study was to investigate the impact of these highly charged bedside phenomena that have both short-term consequences on parent and nurse interactions and long-term consequences on the interactions of the family with the healthcare team. Nurses must acknowledge that these emotional situations require a team effort to keep the families involved with pediatric healthcare services. Because conflicts will likely continue to increase as religious involvement increases, nurses need to arm themselves with information on the various religious doctrines, as well as anticipate the possible conflicts and "storms" that might occur. Best practice will require knowledgeable nurses who can navigate through these difficult situations, while continuing to concentrate on the needs of acutely ill children.

# PARENTS, CLERGY, AND COMMUNITY PERSPECTIVES ON TREATMENT REFUSAL

In the second ethnographic study, the researcher explored the experiences and perspectives of parents, extended family, clergy, and community members. After the investigation of professional nurses' experiences with treatment refusal was complete, the next step of inquiry was family and clergy experiences.

## STUDY #2

### ASSUMPTIONS

1) With increasing church membership and vast cultural diversity expanding in the United States, parental-driven treatment refusal scenarios are likely to increase in pediatric healthcare delivery.

2) Moral distress related to ethical dilemmas has a significant negative impact on pediatric nurses' performance, on healthcare provider and family relationships, and on healthcare provider and clergy relationships. As treatment scenarios continue, and perhaps rise in number, greater acknowledgement and understanding of the dynamics of the scenarios are warranted.

3) Nurses continue to report a lack of knowledge concerning the legal and social factors associated with parental treatment refusal for children during healthcare delivery or illness prevention.

### RESEARCH QUESTIONS

Three research questions were posed to family members (including extended family members), church community members, and clergy. These questions were selected specifically to investigate the perspectives of those most involved in the treatment refusal scenario—those close to or caring for the child.

1) What is the impact of parental religious beliefs on the interactions between family members and the healthcare team during decision-making regarding the medical treatment of the acutely ill child?

2) What are the processes and outcomes of medical treatment refusal, including the loss of guardianship, from the perspectives of the healthcare professionals?

3) What is the impact of mandated treatment against parents' beliefs and wishes on the health state, stress level, and functional status of the healthcare professional involved?

## METHODS

An ethnographic qualitative design was used to investigate treatment refusal and limitation experiences of family members, church community members, and clergy in the greater San Francisco Bay Area. Individuals were sought based on the identified list of 31 religions whose doctrines have been found to influence healthcare treatment decisions for children.

Members of a church were identified as a cultural group based on their unique set of practices, behaviors, and methods of communication. Both in-depth interviews and field notes were taken to capture the cultural phenomenon of parental refusal through the experiences and perspectives of these groups. Seventeen adults participated in a one-time interview, and field notes were taken over the course of 20 weeks. A research assistant was used to help advertise the study purposes and secure participants.

## SAMPLE

Using a convenience, nonprobability sampling procedure, 17 people were recruited for the study. After obtaining written approval from the Institutional Review Board's Committee on Human Research at the University of California, San Francisco, an information packet was prepared and sent to several dozen churches in the greater San Francisco Bay Area. These churches were located via the Internet or phone books, or by networking. Snowball sampling, word-of-mouth, and poster advertising worked most effectively after many unfruitful attempts to locate a diverse representation of the identified churches via mailed information packets.

The sample represented several demographic variables. Fifteen of the 17 participants were female, and 2 of the 3 clergy interviewed were male. Ages ranged from 32 to 74, and all participants interviewed face to face were Caucasian.

## SETTING

Four of the in-depth interviews were conducted by a long-distance telephone call, and 13 were conducted in person. The phone interviews were required because these families were located out of state. Two of the out-of-state families had lost a child as a result of religious beliefs. The face-to-face interviews were conducted in a variety of places, including a library reading room, a park, a hospital waiting room, a coffee shop, and private homes. The environments, although quite diverse, provided ample support for deep sharing and a successful interview.

## INSTRUMENT

The researcher had an interview guide written on a small notepad, but no notes were taken during the interviews. Although all interviews were based on the Institutional Review Board's approved interview guide, the researcher adapted the voicing and the sequence of the questions with each subsequent interview to maximize disclosure and explore each participant's recorded interviews for data saturation. No second interviews were conducted, as each transcribed interview was deemed complete. Field notes were written immediately upon completion of the interviews to document responses, nonverbal communications, and an initial assessment of the discourse.

## INTERVIEWS

Three clergy leaders agreed to be interviewed for the study, each disclosing divergent views. Two of the clergy represented traditional Christian faiths, and one represented a leadership position within the Christian Science faith. Fourteen church members, community members, and individuals were interviewed; church affiliations that were represented included Jehovah's Witnesses ($n=1$), Christian Science ($n=3$), Four Square ($n=1$), and fundamentalist Christian faiths $n=2$). Seven others represented a wide assortment of beliefs, all sharing the common thread of prayer before healthcare, prayer instead of healthcare, or prayer along with healthcare. One mother demonstrated a combination of cultural norms and religious beliefs.

## Procedures

Phone numbers were given directly to the investigator or to a research assistant. Three participants were located via networking. Participants were phoned to set up a location and time for an interview. For the out-of-state telephone interviews, participants were asked to commit to a time when they could have privacy and be undisturbed during the discussion and disclosure.

## Data

Seventeen transcribed interviews were carefully analyzed for content, thematic coding, and narrative analysis. Rich data were collected, and for this initial assessment of the data, three themes were identified.

## Analysis

These themes emerged from the ethnographic data analysis:

1) proud to be a believer;

2) wanting out; and

3) mistrust versus distrust.

## Proud to Be a Believer

Participants described their commitment to their religious frameworks in many ways.

> Being a Christian Scientist means not acknowledging, or not even knowing what disease is. ... You learn to know that there is nothing really wrong with you [disease or illness]. ... Things like headaches and stomachaches do not exist; things like cuts or cancer are going to get better. ... You do not speak of such things.

> My grandmother, a devoted Christian Scientist, she is the one that told me how to pray. She had rectal bleeding for a short time. I slammed my hand in a door and may have broken bones, but she just bandaged me up. ... You know, things are not addressed outside of prayer, just not addressed.

132

My faith is my life; it is how I eat, sleep, and live. My faith does not falter, even during hard times that you would call illness. I do not seek a doctor, as prayer is my center core, my healing, my commitment.

When my mom had me, she was in labor for 2 days. My father said she cried and pounded the mattress all day until I was born. ... She was so proud to be a Christian Scientist; she was trying so hard to be a Christian Scientist; she wanted to stay by herself at home in labor so no one would intervene.

What I want people to know is that it is not easy to balance one's faith now days. ... Yes, we impose on others to keep our faith, but all we want is respect and understanding and compassion. ... It is a hard position to be in, trying to balance our faith with others in the outside world. We just do not consume healthcare like it is going out of style. ... We pray first, always.

I am not on the fringe; I am clear as to what I believe. I just do not want more and more technology influencing my health or my family's health decisions.

Yes, the doctors will make the call to the judge about blood transfusions for our people, but we all are taught to know that this is coming. ... Some believe that their child might be damned for life; others, well, just don't hear that but will not, in good faith, consent.

My brother left the Christian Science church. When he was diagnosed with diabetes, he came back to his faith. ... [He] reaccepted the faith all over again ... no treatment, no nothing. ... He has done very well. He is 50 now.

## WANTING OUT

When I turned 18, I left the faith. I have so many memories of my brother. ... He had migraine headaches and would scream and scream and vomit. ... Yet, there was nothing wrong with him. ... A lot of those things went on when I was growing up.

As soon as he turned 18, he left The Family. ... His broken arm was never set; he never saw a dentist and suffered horribly. ... His mom had melanoma and was never treated. ... The skin was sloughing off her arms. They were strictly Old Testament, not Christ-based, and participated in fasting, severe discipline. ... He never felt loved or supported in his childhood, was never allowed to gather with others. ... [He was] frightened most of the time. ... [He] never played with children outside of the group.

## MISTRUST VERSUS DISTRUST

Some often ask me, "Is it right to impose [our faith] on children?" You know, if in fact there is a choice between life or death, we meet with the parents, and we treat them with respect. We meet with the doctors, and we know we are going to face trouble.

I was never immunized; I never use cheap antibiotics; I do not treat fevers or pain the way you would. ... I know that I am a character, but most of what doctors do for your kids is harmful and destructive. I used compresses and lymphatic raking on my kids; they grew up just fine without [doctors]. (no church affiliation)

## SUMMARY OF FINDINGS

The participants in the ethnographic interviews were either very descriptive in their faith and commitment to their beliefs or were graphic in their discussions of "getting out." Members of one family described how their faith and decisions about their children's health were regrettable. One daughter described her mother's life as "ruined" by her beliefs. Still others remain steadfast, faithful, and true to their religious beliefs, describing how prayer has been a valuable tool for health and well-being.

The data, although limited by the number of participants and the restricted geographical location, showed the unique perspectives of the parents. Both religious beliefs and cultural beliefs are broad areas requiring extensive investigation. No two families represented exactly the same experiences, priorities, or desires for their children during the refusal or limitation of treatment scenario. This demonstrates further the complexity of treatment refusal and the need for careful consideration to the uniqueness of each family's belief structure.

# IMPLICATIONS FOR CARE

Pediatric healthcare professionals must conduct an assessment of family beliefs if consenting or adhering to treatment is questionable. Based on the evidence presented by the two ethnographic investigations in this chapter, implementation of the following decision-making and interventional steps during refusal or limitation scenarios is recommended. Post this list where it can be accessed when situations arise:

1) Immediately identify delays in parents seeking care, consenting for care, refusing diagnostics for children, or not following prescribed nursing care or medical interventions.

2) Identify unattended symptom experiences (pain, nausea, sleep disturbances, fatigue, emotional distress, or dyspnea), and determine the underlying belief structures that are influencing parents to ignore or not treat the symptoms.

3) Assess the family's understanding of the severity of the untreated condition.

4) Communicate immediately the limitation, delay, or refusal of treatment to the interdisciplinary team. Elicit group participation and organization.

5) Investigate and educate the team on specifics found in the literature or online concerning the religious or cultural group's belief systems.

6) Offer to bring in and meet with clergy, elders, or other parishioners to provide support for the family and further educate the healthcare team.

7) Establish a culture of trust while communicating the priority status of the child's well-being.

8) Apply the principles of family-centered care (enabling and empowering) to each family member, ensuring the goal of care is centered on holding the family as the child's constant, and respect the family's need to apply religious or cultural beliefs or practices.

9) Ensure the safety of the child at all times. Seek interventions from social workers and request temporary legal guardianship if required, but only as a last resort after family conferences and negotiations are complete.

10) Provide lifesaving, life-prolonging medical treatments as needed. Provide symptom management and support the child during the process.

11) Maintain a respectful relationship with the immediate and extended family to ensure ongoing continuation of care.

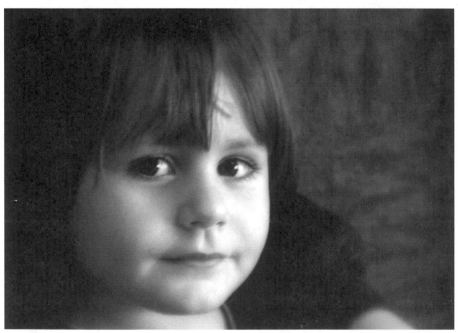

*Photo by Simona Balint. www.sxc.hu/profile/simmbarb*

# REFERENCES

American Academy of Pediatrics Committee on Bioethics. (1988). Religious exemptions from child abuse. *Pediatrics, 81*(1), 169-171.

American Academy of Pediatrics Committee on Bioethics. (1995). Informed consent, parental permission, and assent in pediatric practice. *Pediatrics, 95*, 314-317.

American Academy of Pediatrics Committee on Bioethics. (1997). Religious objections of medical care. *Pediatrics, 99*, 279-280.

Anderson, G.R. (1983). Medicine vs. religion: The case of Jehovah's Witnesses. *Health and Social Work, 8*, 31-38.

Appelbaum, P., & Roth, L. (1983). Patients who refuse treatment in medical hospitals. *Journal of the American Medical Association, 250*(10), 1296-1301.

Associated Jehovah's Witnesses for Reform on Blood (AJWRB). (n.d.). Retrieved July 24, 2006, from http://www.ajwrb.org

Bodnaruk, Z.M., Wong, C.J., & Thomas, M.J.. (2004). Meeting the clinical challenge of care for Jehovah's Witnesses. *Transfusion Medicine Reviews, 18*(2), 105-116.

Bromley, D.G., & Melton, J.G. (Eds.). (2002). *Cults, Religion and Violence*. Cambridge, UK: Cambridge University Press.

Byrd, R.C. (1998). Positive therapeutic effects of intercessory prayer in a coronary care unit population. *Southern Medical Journal, 81*(7), 826-829.

Catlin, A. (1997). Commentary of Johnny's story: Transfusing a Jehovah's Witness. *Pediatric Nursing, 23*(3), 289-291, 317.

CHILD, Inc. Children's healthcare is a legal duty. (2006, July). Retrieved May 18, 2006, from http://www.childrenshealthcare.org

Clutter, L. (2005). Spiritual issues in children's health-care settings. In J.A. Rollins, R. Bolig., & C.C. Mahan (Eds.), *Meeting children's psychosocial needs across the health-care continuum*, 351-420. Austin, TX: Pro-Ed, Inc.

Corley, M., Elswick, R., & Gorman, M. (2001). Development and evaluation of a moral distress scale. *Journal of Advanced Nursing, 33*(2), 250-256.

Cushing, M. (1982). Whose best interest? Parents vs. child rights. *American Journal of Nursing, 82*(2), 313-314.

Denzin, N.K., & Lincoln, Y.S. (2000). *Handbook of qualitative research* (2nd ed.). Thousand Oaks, CA: Sage.

Dodes, I. (1987). Suffer the little children...: Toward a judicial recognition of duty of reasonable care owed children by religious faith healers. *Hofstra Law Review, 16,* 165-190.

Dominican University. (2001). *Issues on spirituality and research lecture series.* San Rafael, CA: Author.

Dusek, J., Astin, J., Hibberd, P., & Krucoff, M. (2003). Healing prayer outcomes studies: Consensus recommendations. *Alternative Therapies, 9*(3), A44-A53.

Dwyer, J. (1996). The children we abandon: Religious exemptions to child welfare and education laws as denials of equal protection to children of religious objectors. *North Carolina Law Review, 74,* 1321-1478.

Dyer, J. (2000). *Faith healing and dying kids.* Retrieved July 25, 2006, from http://www.boulderweekly.com/archive/030101/dyertimes.html

Eddy, M.B. (1875). *Science and health with key to the scriptures* (1971 ed.). Boston: Christian Science Publishing Society.

Eddy, M.B. (1925). *Prose works other than science and health.* Boston: Christian Science Publishing Society.

Evans, T., & Trotter, E. (2006, July 13). State settles in death of boy taken from mother. *The Indianapolis Star.* Retrieved July 17, 2006, from http://nl.newsbank.com/nl-search/we/Archives.

The First Church of Christ, Scientist. (2006). *Publications and broadcasts.* Retrieved July 25, 2006, from http://www.tfccs.com/media/

Flannery, E. (1995). One advocate's viewpoint: Conflicts and tension in the Baby K case. *Journal of Law, Medicine and Ethics, 23*(1), 7-12.

Foreman, D.M. (1999). The family rule: Framework for obtaining ethical consent. *Journal of Medical Ethics, 25*(6), 491-496.

Fost, N. (1981). Ethical issues in the treatment of critically ill newborns. *Pediatric Annals, 10*(10), 16-52.

Fox, V. (1990). Caught between religion and medicine. *AORN Journal, 52*(1), 131-146.

Gallup Organization. (2006). *Gallup poll on religion in the United States.* Princeton, NJ: Author.

Glover, R.J., & Rushton, C. (1995). Introducing: From Baby Doe to Baby K. *Evolving Challenges in Pediatric Ethics, 23*(1), 5-8.

Habler, O. (2005). Blood safety: Artificial oxygen carriers offer an alternative to red blood cell transfusion. *Obesity, Fitness & Wellness Week.* 3 December 2005. Retrieved 21 August 2006 from: http://www.newsrx.com/newsletters/Obesity,-Fitness-and-Wellness-Week/2005-12-03/1203200533396OW.html

Hammersley, M., & Atkinson, P. (1995). *Ethnography: Principles in practice* (2nd ed.). London: Routledge.

Hanna, D.R., & Roy, C. (2001). Roy adaptation model and perspectives on the family. *Nursing Science Quarterly, 14*, 10-13.

Heller, J. (1998). *It's freedom vs. responsibility.* Retrieved August 19, 2004, from www.sptimes.com/TampaBay.

Hockenberry, M. (2004). *Wong's essentials of pediatric nursing.* St. Louis, MO: Mosby.

Humber, J.M., & Almeder, R.F. (2000). *Is there a duty to die?* Totowa, NJ: Humana Press.

International Cultic Studies Association. (2005). *Cultic studies: Information about cults and psychological manipulation.* Retrieved May 18, 2006, from http://www.csj.org/

Jameton, A. (1993). Dilemmas of moral distress: Moral responsibility and nursing practice. *AWHONN's Clinical Issues in Perinatal and Women's Health Nursing, 4*, 542-551.

Janofsky, M. (2001). *Colorado children's deaths rekindle debate on religion.* Retrieved August 29, 2004, from http://www.sullivan-county.com

Kondos, E. (1992). The law and Christian Science healing for children: A pathfinder. *Legal Reference Services Quarterly, 12*(1), 5-71.

Kopelman, L., Irons, T., & Kopelman, A. (1988). Neonatologists judge the "Baby Doe" regulations. *The New England Journal of Medicine, 318*(11), 677-683.

Kostinchuk, D. (2001). *Faith healing: Child abuse, torture and homicide.* Retrieved July 28, 2006, from http://www.positiveatheism.org/mail/eml9074.htm

Lantos, J., & Miles, S. (1989). Autonomy in adolescent medicine: A framework for decision about life-sustaining treatment. *Journal of Adolescent Healthcare, 10*(6), 460-468.

Larabee, M. (1998). *The battle over faith healing: When prayer pre-empts medical care, prosecutors nationwide struggle to respect parents' freedoms while protecting children's lives.* Retrieved summer 2005 from http://www.rickross.com/

Lawry, K., Slomka, J., & Goldfarb, J. (1996). What went wrong: Multiple perspectives on an adolescent's decision to refuse blood transfusions. *Clinical Pediatrics, 35*(6), 317-322.

LeCompte, M., & Schensul, J. (1999). *The ethnographer's tool kit.* Walnut Creek, CA: AltaMira Press.

Leininger, M., & McFarland, M.R. (2002). *Transcultural nursing: Concepts, theories, research and practice* (3rd ed.). Hightstown, NJ: McGraw-Hill.

Lerner, M. (1994). *Choices in healing: Integrating the best of conventional and complementary approaches to cancer.* Retrieved July 18, 2006, from http://www.commonweal.org

Levin, J. (1994). Religion and health: Is there an association, is it valid, and is it causal? *Social Science Medicine, 38*(11), 1475-1482.

Levin, J. (2006, July 13). *Jeff Levin, PhD.* Retrieved July 28, 2006, from http://religionandhealth.com/

Linnard-Palmer, L., & Kools, S. (2004). Parents' refusal of medical treatment based on religious and/or cultural beliefs: The law, ethical principles, and clinical implications. *Journal of Pediatric Nursing, 19*(5), 351-356.

Linnard-Palmer, L., & Kools, S. (2005). Parents' refusal of medical treatment for cultural or religious beliefs: An ethnographic study of healthcare professionals' experiences. *Journal of Pediatric Oncology Nursing, 22*(1), 48-57.

Lipson, J., Dibble, S., & Minarik, P. (1996). *Culture and nursing care: A pocket guide.* San Francisco: UCSF Nursing Press.

Macklin, R. (1988). The inner workings of an ethics committee: Latest battle over Jehovah's Witnesses. *Hasting Center Report, 18*(1), 15-20.

Mann, M., Votto, J., Kambe, J., & McNamee, M. (1992). Management of severely anemic patient who refuses transfusion: Lessons learned during the care of a Jehovah Witness. *Annals of Internal Medicine, 117*(2), 1043-1048.

Massachusetts Citizens for Children. (1992). *Death by religious exemption.* Retrieved July 27, 2006, from http://masskids.org/dbre/index.html

Meyer, J. (1996, June 21). The spiritual-healing alternative. *The Denver Post.*

Migden, D., & Braen, G. (1998). The Jehovah's Witness blood refusal care: Ethical and medicolegal considerations for emergency physicians. *Academic Emergency Medicine, 5,* 815-824.

Monopoli, P. (1991). Allocating the costs of parental free exercise: Striking a balance between sincere religious belief and a child's right to medical treatment. *Pepperdine Law Review, 18,* 319-352.

Muramoto, O. (1998). Medical ethics in the treatment of Jehovah's Witnesses. *Archives of Internal Medicine, 158*(10), 1155-1156.

Muramoto, O. (1999). Recent developments in medical care of Jehovah's Witnesses. *World Journal of Medicine, 5*(170), 297-301.

Murray, J. (2004, April 6). Parents: Boy grew sicker after removal from home. *The Indianapolis Star.* Retrieved July 17, 2006, from http://nl.newsbank.com/nl-search/we/Archives.

Neeley, G.S. (1998). Legal and ethical dilemmas surrounding prayer as a method of alternative healing for children. In J.M. Humber & R.F. Almeder (Eds.), *Alternative medicine and ethics,* 163-194. Totowa, NJ: Humana Press.

New England Institute of Religious Research. (n.d.). The body of Christ: Descent from benign Bible study to destructive cult. Retrieved May 30, 2006, from http://neirr.org/AttleboroHistoryNew.htm

Ontario Consultants on Religious Tolerance. (n.d.). Retrieved summer 2003 from http://www.religioustolerance.org

Overbay, J.D. (1996). Parental participation in treatment decisions for pediatric oncology and intensive care unit patients. *Dimensions of Critical Care Nursing, 15*(1), 16-24.

Paris, J. (1982). Terminating treatment for newborns: A theological perspective. *Law, Medicine and Health Care, 10*(3), 120-124, 144.

Paris, J., & Bell, A. (1993). Guarantee my child will be "normal" or stop all treatment. *Journal of Perinatology, 13*(6), 469-472.

People v. New York, Peirson. (1903).

Perkin, R.M., Young, T., Freier, M.C., Allen, J., & Orr, R.D. (1997). Stress and distress in pediatric nurses: Lessons from Baby K. *American Journal of Critical Care; 6*(3), 225-232.

Prince v. Massachusetts, 321 158 (U.S. 1943-1944).

Purssell, E. (1995). Listening to children: Medical treatment and consent. *Journal of Advanced Nursing, 21*(4), 623-624.

Quintero, C. (1993). Blood administration in pediatric Jehovah's Witnesses. *Pediatric Nursing, 19*(1), 46-48.

Reaves, J. (2001). *Freedom of religion or state-sanctioned child abuse?* Retrieved summer 2005 from http://www.time.com

Rhodes, A. (1995). Guardianship and the refusal of treatment. *Maternal Child Nursing, 20*(2), 109.

Rhodes, A.M., & Miller, R.D. (1984). *Nursing and the law.* Rockville, MD: Aspen Systems Corp.

Rick A. Ross Institute of New Jersey. (n.d., p. 6). Retrieved summer 2003 from http://www.rickross.com/

Rosaldo, R. (1993). *Culture and truth: The remaking of social analysis* (2nd ed.). Boston: Beacon.

Ruccione, K., Kramer, R., Moore, I., & Perin, G. (1991). Informed consent for treatment of childhood cancer: Factors affecting parents' decision making. *Journal of Pediatric Oncology Nursing, 8*(3), 112-121.

Seth, A., & Swan, R. (1998). Child fatalities from religion-motivated medical neglect. *Pediatrics, 101*(4), 625-629.

Shepherd, B. (n.d.) *Deborah Elizabeth Shepherd, 1974-1983: Where were you, Lord?* (para. 11-13). Retrieved July 28, 2006, from http://www.geocities.com/Heartland/Woods/1327/

Spahn, D.R., Kocian, R. (2005). Artificial oxygen carriers: Status in 2005. *Current Pharmaceutical Design.* 2005;11(31):4099-114.

Stubbs, J.R. (2006). Alternatives to blood transfusion in critically ill: Erythropoietin. *Critical Care Medicine.* May; 34 (5 Supplement). 5106-0.

Sundin-Huard, D., & Fahy, K. (1999). Moral distress, advocacy and burnout: Theorizing the relationships. *International Journal of Nurse Practitioners, 5*(1), 8-13.

Sung, K.C., et al. (2006). In pediatric cardiac surgery, hydroxyethyl starch is a safe alternative for volume replacement. *Obesity, Fitness & Wellness Week.* 25 March 2006. Retrieved 21 August 2006 from http://www.newsrx.com/newsletters/Obesity,-Fitness-and-Wellness-Week/2006-03-25/032520063331524OW.html

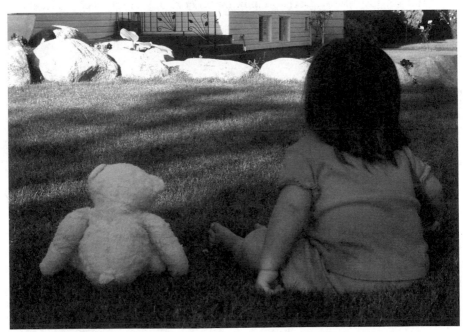

*Photo by Adrian Yer. www.sxc.hu/profile/vancity197*

Swan, R. (1997). Children, medicine, religion, and the law. *Advances in Pediatrics, 44,* 491-544.

Swan, R. (2000, November). When faith fails children. *The Humanist, 16*(6).

Talbot, N.A. (1983). The position of the Christian Science Church. *The New England Journal of Medicine, 309*(26), 1641-1644.

Thurkauf, G. (1989). Understanding the beliefs of Jehovah's Witnesses. *Focus on Critical Care, 16*(3), 199-204.

Tierney, W., Weinberger, M., Greene, J., & Studdard, A. (1984). Jehovah's Witnesses and blood transfusion: Physicians attitudes and legal precedent. *Southern Medical Journal, 77*(4), 473-477.

Trotter, E. (2004, August 19). Boy's death stumps officials. *The Indianapolis Star.* Retrieved July 17, 2006, from http://nl.newsbank. com/nl-search/we/Archives

Vercillo, A.P., & Duprey, S.V. (1988). Jehovah's Witnesses and the transfusion of blood products. *New York State Journal of Medicine, 88,* 493-494.

Watchko, J.F. (1983). Decision making on critically ill infants by parents. *American Journal of Diseases of Children, 137,* 795-798.

Wong, D. (2004) Essentials of Pediatric Nursing. Lippincott.

# Epilogue

Nurses, physicians, and related pediatric healthcare professionals are in a unique position to offer support to families who are experiencing the critical dilemma of wanting prayer in lieu of medical care, or wishing to limit medical care based on cultural or religious doctrine. Although the healthcare professionals involved may not agree with the application of parental cultural or religious beliefs on children's medical decision-making, and may proceed with securing state guardianship and mandated treatment, families deserve respect and a voice. They deserve the opportunity to explain their beliefs and preferences, alone or in the presence of their clergy or elder, when time is not dictated by the critical status of the child's condition. Pediatric healthcare professionals can minimize the stress, fear, anxiety, and possible anger of family members by demonstrating an understanding of diverse beliefs and allowing time, whenever safe and possible, for each family member to disclose his or her concerns and belief systems.

Members of healthcare professions who encounter families of diverse cultural and religious backgrounds must be knowledgeable about legal and ethical principles, as well as basic foundations of various religious doctrines. Healthcare professionals can be better prepared to participate in treatment decisions if they are well-versed in a variety of literature (and how to retrieve the literature) and are aware of the many viable perspectives on treatment refusal.

Because of the lack of research in the area of parental treatment refusal, further investigations are warranted across all healthcare professions. Whether one is a pharmacist, physical or occupational therapist, nurse, physician, or social worker, further investigations on the processes and outcomes across the nation, representing various state-based exemptions, must continue.

It is important to note that there is a reality to spiritual abuse. Not all of the 31 organizations mentioned in this book adhere to doctrines of such magnitude that one can consider the teachings dangerous and the followers abused, but there are cults with such powerful influences over the followers that they can be interpreted as abusive. The church-mandated delay or refusal to seek medical care and treatment for children should be considered an example of how influential cult teaching can be.

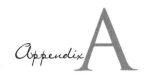

# GUIDELINES FOR STAFF FACING PARENTAL REFUSAL OF PEDIATRIC TREATMENT

Suggested steps to take:

1) Ensure the child is safe, cared for, and under nursing or healthcare supervision at all times. Assess for changes in clinical status that may occur as a result of the child not receiving immediate nursing or medical care (such as a STAT blood product transfusion or needed medical intervention).

2) Maintain respectful contact with all family members.

3) Identify the primary decision-maker within the family structure.

4) Explain the necessary treatments or diagnostic tests needed.

5) Request the name of the family's church, organization, or cultural group whose teachings or doctrines are influencing consent or refusal to participate in the medical treatment or diagnostic procedures.

6) Contact the primary physician or primary care provider and explain the family's concerns about the ordered treatments and the specifics of the refusal request, including the name of the church, organization, or cultural group.

7) Upon the physician's or primary care provider's request, ask the family for names and phone numbers of clergy, elders, or contact people associated with the religion, faith, or cultural group from which they want support and/or assistance.

8) Notify social services or follow the institution's policy and procedures for contacting appropriate hospital/clinic administrators. This may include a member of upper management and administration, as well as a member of the institution's ethics committee.

9) Request a conference for the family and health care professionals.

10) Have a colleague assist with a computer search for information of the church, organization, or cultural group. Print and place this information in the medical chart.

11) Continually assess the probability of the family leaving "against medical advice."

12) Provide support and respect and keep in constant communication with the family. Explain what is happening, why, and who is involved.

13) Carefully document all assessments, calls, and interventions. Include contact information on family members and their church, organization, or cultural group.

14) If a child protective agency is engaged, make sure all charting is accurate and thorough. Fill out appropriate forms and make duplicates of medical records.

15) Continue to be the family's support system and be factual, non-judgmental, and straightforward in all communications. Keep explaining that your priority is the well-being of the child.

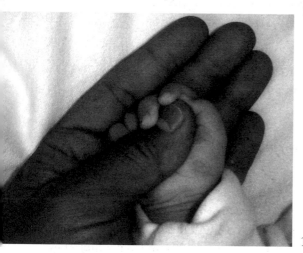

16) Attempt, when safe and possible, to include church members, faith practices, cultural practices, prayer sessions, or any safe and appropriate practices that the family may request in the plan of care. Check with the institution's supervisor if a practice is potentially unsafe or prohibited (such as candle burning).

17) After the refusal situation is over, debrief with professional colleagues so that all involved feel educated and enlightened by the experience.

# RESOURCES

## SENTENCE AND KEYWORD SUGGESTIONS FOR INTERNET SEARCHING:

This section presents suggested search sentences or keywords for locating information via the Internet. Web links can and do change frequently; thus, it's most beneficial to follow the suggested search patterns listed below by using any Internet search engine, such as Google, Yahoo, Dogpile, Lycos, AltaVista, or MSN.

- Rick Ross (www.rickross.com)
- A Pastor Deplores Spiritual Abuse
- Ontario Consultants on Religious Tolerance
- Jan Groenveld's Links (http://www.cultinfo.org.au/linkbook.htm)
- Unhealthy Influences Within the Church
- The Next Billy Graham? Or a UPC cultist?
- Atlanta Christian Apologetics Project
- Cults and Spiritually Abusive Churches
- Answers in Action: Fighting Falsehood
- Recovering From Spiritual Abuse
- Families Against Cults
- Limits of Pastoral Authority
- Vicarious Atonement—Is It Real?
- Jehovah's Witnesses Child Abuse
- Counter-Cult Links and Resources
- Walk Away; Ex-fundamentalists

- Survivors of Spiritual Abuse
- Christian Anti-Cult Outreach
- ReFocus Page
- FACTNet
- UNI.CC
- R.E.S.T.
- AFF

## PRINT BOOK RECOMMENDATIONS:

http://www.rickross.com/reference/books/reading_list.html

*Faith Beyond Faith Healing,* by Kimberly Winston (Paraclete Press, 2002)

Search online library or bookseller databases for "spiritual healing."

## OTHER RESOURCES:

1) Watchtower Society publications

2) Christian Science Reading Rooms

3) *Born in Zion,* by former Registered Nurse Carol Balizet, who promotes Christian home births, and believes that medical care is linked with pagan witchcraft

4) Hernandez-Arriaga, J., Aldana-Valenzuela, C., & Iserson, K. (2001). Jehovah's Witnesses and medical practice in Mexico: Religious freedom, parens patriae, and the right to life. *Cambridge Quarterly of Healthcare Ethics, 10,* 47-52.

5) The Islamic Medical Association of North America. (www.imana.org)

6) Associated Jehovah's Witnesses for Reform on Blood (www.ajwrb.org)

7) Elena Kondos's article on "The Law and Christian Science Healing for Children: A Pathfinder" (1991) in *Legal Reference Services Quarterly 12*(1), 5-71 detailing descriptions of exemptions, laws, beliefs, and resources for further study.

8) Rita Swan's article, "Children, Medicine, Religion and the Law" (1997). *Advances in Pediatrics, 44,* 491-544.

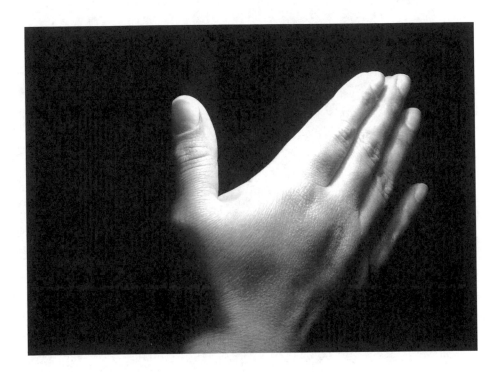

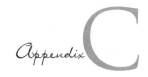

# FIVE REASONS FOR COURTS TO OVERRIDE A PATIENT'S RIGHT TO REFUSE MEDICAL TREATMENT

The following have been noted within several U.S. laws as reasons for courts to intervene and order treatment:

1) preservation of life when the patient's condition is curable;

2) protection of the patient's dependents, especially minor children;

3) prevention of irrational self-destruction;

4) preservation of ethical integrity of healthcare providers; and

5) protection of the public health and other interests.

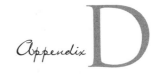

*Appendix* D

# REASONS FOR PARENTAL DECISIONS TO REFUSE MEDICAL TREATMENTS

There are numerous, powerful reasons behind parental decisions to refuse or limit medical treatment. The following list was condensed from health science and related literature of the past 21 years.

1) Religious frameworks concerning preference for prayer over traditional medical treatments or prior to any traditional medical care were found nationally and internationally.

2) Religious frameworks concerning limits on interventions such as various blood and blood product transfusion therapies, specialized diet therapies, or diagnostics have been found across America.

3) Ambiguous consenting procedures by healthcare professionals seeking parental approval and signature for medical treatments, diagnostics, or other procedures can lead to refusal to sign consent forms. Often, healthcare providers try to rush the process for obtaining consent for diagnostics, treatments, transfusions, or surgeries, leading parents to refuse or delay consent. This rush is often related to the hectic interdisciplinary schedule of pediatric hospital departments.

4) Conflicting or ambiguous sources of information on treatment decisions are not unusual. Because of the vast array of technology, it is not uncommon for parents to seek second or third opinions. This can delay consent or treatments.

5) Influences on the access to sophisticated medical technology can lead to fears, confusion, and delays in treatment consent.

6) Pressures during the treatment decision-making time frame can occur. Some religious or cultural practices warrant counsel by church elders, high-level church representatives, or tribal leaders, which in turn causes treatment delays.

7) Conscientious objectors to medical care or treatment exist. Some people simply do not trust or wish to apply modern, standardized medical care. Many in this category are not affiliated with any particular cultural or religious group. Some may feel that procedures are overlapping, or repeated measures are just not warranted. Sometimes they are right and sometimes they are not. This mistrust of medical procedures may add to the confusion.

8) Use of alternative medicine modalities rather than Western medical practices has become commonplace. With the rising number of Americans who use complementary, alternative, or integrative treatments, parental desires to apply various nontraditional healing methods are escalating.

9) Parental relationships with other siblings can become strained or compromised. The sacrifice of family life (quality of life) during the demands of care for the child requiring treatment may be perceived to be too great. In other words, families may say "no" to a complex and expensive treatment for one child so that the quality of life of the family as a whole is not changed or is minimally impacted.

10) Cost in dollars and loss of employment or inability to maintain employment during care for the ill child can cause parents to refuse treatment.

11) Mental capacity of parents making treatment decisions may influence consenting procedures or treatment decision-making. Illiteracy, lower educational levels, and poor comprehension abilities can influence whether or not a parent readily consents for medical treatments.

12) Pressures and emotional turmoil during treatment decisions may be too great.

13) Mental capabilities of children for whom treatment decisions are being made may influence parents' treatment decisions.

14) Issues concerning best interest for the child may influence consenting procedures.

15) Concerns of quality of life for the child after complex medical treatments with few known positive outcomes may influence parental decisions.

(Information summarized by Overbay, 1996; Paris & Bell, 1993; Rhodes, 1995; Ruccione, Kramer, Moore, & Perin, 1991.)

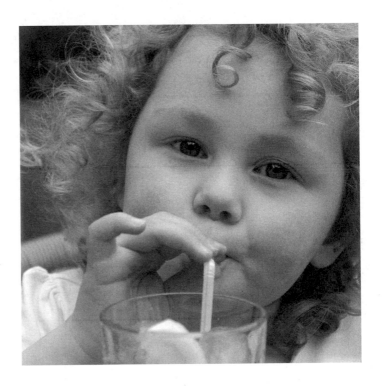

# RELIGIOUS GROUPS CURRENTLY IDENTIFIED AS INFLUENTIAL ON HEALTHCARE TREATMENT DECISIONS

The following list includes 31 religious groups found in the current literature whose doctrines, or teachings, have been noted to influence decisions about children's healthcare:

1) Jehovah's Witnesses

2) Christian Science

3) The Church of the First Born

4) Christian Catholic Church (Not affiliated with the Roman Catholic Church)

5) Faith Assembly

6) Followers of Christ

7) End Time Ministries

8) The Believers' Fellowship

9) Faith Temple Doctoral Church of Christ in God

10) The Source

11) Christ Miracle Healing Center

12) "No Name" Fellowship

13) The Fellowship

14) Faith Tabernacle Congregation

15) 1st Century Gospel

16) Pentecostal Church

17) Evangelistic Healers

18) Jesus Through Jon and Judy

19) Wiccans (people who identify themselves as Witches; not a religious order)

20) Four Square Church

21) Christ Assembly

22) The Church of God of the Union Assembly

23) Church of God Chapel

24) Northeast Kingdom Community Church

25) True Followers of Christ

26) Faith Cathedral Assembly

27) Living Word Assembly of God

28) Traveling Ministries Everyday Church

29) Bible Readers Fellowship

30) The Body (a.k.a. The Body of Christ)

31) Oregon-based Christ Church

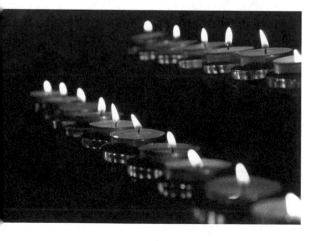

# SECTS AND CULTS: ADDITIONAL INFORMATION

David Kostinchuk (2001) offers brief examples of a number of the above religions. In describing their beliefs, he sheds light on how they receive public awareness. He titles them the "players" and offers this information with numerous helpful references:

1)  The Bible Readers Fellowship, an evangelical group located in California, does not report or record births or deaths as required by state law. The group supports avoidance of all medical treatments.

2)  Members of the End Time Ministries sect hold faith healing as a high belief. They reject medical interventions for their children and do not allow healthcare professionals to be present at their births.

3)  Members of the Oregon-based Christ Church believe in the power of prayer as a cure for medical conditions. They prefer to use anointing oils and "laying on of hands" rather than traditional medical interventions, even for their children.

4)  Many Pentecostal sects also believe in "laying on of hands" rather than seeking medical attention for their members (including children).

5)  Faith Tabernacle Congregation Church members believe they can be cured of sickness by the prayers of "true believers." Members who seek medical care are seen by some members as turning their backs on God and their faith.

6) The sovereign power of God to heal is the central belief of followers of the General Assembly Church of the First Born.

7) Members of the Faith Tabernacle Church are encouraged to follow what the group sees as God's will, including the notion that God's will is to not seek medical treatment, even for church members' children.

# INDEX

# R